YOU ARE GETTING SLEEPY

Lifestyle-Based
Solutions for Insomnia

Paul Glovinsky PhD
& Arthur Spielman PhD

DIVERSIONBOOKS

D0011638

Diversion Books
A Division of Diversion Publishing Corp.
443 Park Avenue South, Suite 1008
New York, New York 10016
www.DiversionBooks.com

For more information, email info@diversionbooks.com

First Diversion Books edition July 2017.
Print ISBN: 978-1-68230-822-6
eBook ISBN: 978-1-68230-821-9

For Arthur Spielman, PhD, and Aaron Sher, MD

I met both of you practically the same minute, on a Thursday late in 1979. A second-year grad student, sitting in my first case conference at Montefiore in the Bronx, I was bowled over by two successive waves of fervor. Your shared initials should have tipped me off: not just my working, but my waking hours would be awash in enthusiasm for Anything Sleep. Your distinct means of pursuing understanding—the intrepid intuitions of the theorist, the meticulous probes of the surgeon—together yielded a collegial yin and yang. I threw in my lot with two consummate clinicians, each with a passion for research, each with a great heart. Art and Aaron, I will be forever thankful our work, and our lives, intertwined.

TABLE OF CONTENTS

CHAPTER THREE:
Are You Fatigued Instead of Sleepy?

CHAPTER FOUR:
Are You Too Depressed to Sleep?

CHAPTER FIVE:
Are You Too Anxious to Sleep? 116

CHAPTER SIX:
Are You Too Out of Sync to Sleep? 142

CHAPTER SEVEN: Are You Too Dependent on Medication for Sleep?

Getting Sleepy is the Way to Sleep

Why read a book about getting sleepy? Sleepiness is a state no one aspires to. Nearly all would agree that getting sleepy is just an irritant, a side effect of being awake too long. It's something to be ignored for as long as possible, or "pushed through" if necessary. Those of you reading this book are no doubt hoping for more sleep—but certainly not for more sleepiness! In fact, some of you might say you are plenty sleepy already. By day, sleepiness saps your vitality and interferes with your functioning. By night it taunts you by refusing to give way to sleep itself.

Some of you, on the other hand, may be perplexed by your *lack* of sleepiness. How can you be so hyper, so wired, when you hardly sleep at all? Sure, you'd like to be able to wind down—but *all* the way down, to sleep. Sleepiness you can do without.

Our response to this anticipated chorus of protest is twofold: First, at the risk of being pedantic we'll note that to be "sleepy," in the full sense of the word, implies more than just being drowsy or in need of sleep. It also carries the promise of being "inclined to sleep" or "ready to sleep."

Seen from this vantage, sleepiness is the threshold of sleep. Moreover, it is a portal that can be reached through effort. The willpower required to keep a later bedtime, for example, may lead to sleepiness, as might the mental exercises required to keep a pressing problem at bay until morning. Once you are sleepy, however, you cannot push yourself any further. Poised between the two great states of wakefulness and sleep, you may just have to linger on that threshold for a while. So long as you remain sleepy, sleep will soon enough be ready to receive you.

This appeal to the full sense of *sleepy* is not just semantics. The Multiple Sleep Latency Test (MSLT), long the sleep field's gold standard when it comes to measuring sleepiness, is thought of as gauging "the propensity to sleep." In the MSLT people are essentially put to bed in a dark, quiet room (albeit with lots of monitoring equipment attached), asked to close their eyes, and sleep. Those who fall asleep quickly are officially deemed "sleepier" than those who do not. So you may be fatigued, exhausted, hyperaroused, exasperated, or many other things as you lie in bed unable to sleep, *but you are not really sleepy.*

Next we'll be realists. The second reason we suggest you aim for sleepiness, rather than sleep itself, cuts to the chase of the problem of insomnia: there is no treatment, behavioral or pharmacological, that will ensure that you sleep well on a given night. We emphasized in our 2006 book *The Insomnia Answer* that sleep can be a maddeningly elusive goal: the harder you try to fall asleep, the less likely you are to be successful. The upshot is that sleep cannot be forced. Ultimately, it must come to you.

The metaphor we used to convey this notion was that of surfers who paddle out into the ocean to "catch the wave." They certainly don't go chasing after it. However, surfers still have to make *some* effort as they position themselves for a good ride. They may need to adjust their approach, for example, to changing weather and shoreline conditions. Similarly, you can learn to position yourself for a good night's sleep. Here is a task where all your hard effort will actually pay off, for you *can* learn how to get sleepy. And getting sleepy, in the full sense of the word, is the most reliable way to get to sleep.

• • •

Many of you are already being treated for insomnia with medications or cognitive behavioral therapies, or have tried these interventions in the past with limited success. You may be wondering how the recommendations you will encounter in this book fit in with (and differ from!) what you have already done.

Our objective in writing this book is to offer a more individualized approach, taking into account the particular challenges that stand in *your* way to better sleep. This includes setting the stage with specific preparatory steps, and then emphasizing different treatment components, depending on what is predisposing you to sleep poorly. In addition, we will address maladaptive behavioral and cognitive responses that are more likely to appear in your personal repertoire.

Just as we take a comprehensive history on every new patient we work with, trying to get a good sense of who that person is before formulating an individualized treatment plan, our hope here is that we can rely on your ability to spot yourself in our chapter headings to help guide the formulation of a more nuanced set of recommendations. Some of the concerns tackled in the chapters you choose may seem awfully idiosyncratic to readers who recognize their symptoms in other parts of the book.

So for those of you who have already been treated for insomnia without much success, we ask that you keep an open mind regarding your prospects for better sleep. Whether these previous treatments were of a general nature, such as deep breathing exercises, or the sleep-specific therapies of Cognitive Behavioral Treatment for Insomnia (CBT-I), what may have been missing from the mix was adequate allowance for the particular factors predisposing *you* to insomnia.

If you are currently relying on sleeping pills, this book should still prove beneficial. The tailored cognitive and behavioral interventions you will encounter here can work synergistically with medication to improve sleep. That is, they can help your medicine yield better sleep on a given night, and also maintain its effectiveness over longer durations of treatment.

Our approach fosters collaboration between you and your medication, so you can at least share credit for the sleep you get. This is no small achievement, as regaining confidence in your natural ability to sleep should be a key long-term objective. Ultimately, it may allow you and your prescribing provider to lower the dosage of your sleep medication, or taper you off altogether.

So now we may return to, and expand upon, our original question. Since numerous books explaining CBT-I—a proven, evidence-based treatment—are already on the shelf, and our goal is to optimize that treatment by taking your personal characteristics into account, why introduce a focus on *getting sleepy*?

Well, just as we have come to realize that getting sleepy is the best way to get to sleep, we have also grown to appreciate that the major components of CBT-I as well as many ancillary insomnia treatments really work *to the extent they promote sleepiness at bedtime.* That is, they position poor sleepers to catch the wave of sleep. Whether it is strengthening adaptive associations to the bed and bedroom through stimulus control instructions, reining in a racing mind with guided imagery, addressing dysfunctional thinking through cognitive therapy, or heightening the sleep drive through sleep restriction therapy, these interventions all aim to bring about sleepiness at the right time and place.

If sleepiness can be seen as a common entry into sleep, the paths we take to reach that jumping-off place and the obstacles we must surmount to get there are quite varied. This should not come as a surprise: We all sleep in different environments, constrained by different schedules. Our brains vary in their need for sleep, in their ability to fall and stay sleep, and in their natural preference for when to sleep. Our waking hours, too, are shaped by differences in thinking, behaviors, relationships, beliefs, attitudes, and moods.

All these differences, operating night and day, affect our readiness for sleep.

This multiplicity poses a significant clinical challenge: while numerous routes lead to sleepiness, many more hit a roadblock, circling back to wakefulness and frustration. Fortunately, a better understanding of who you are, and what you "bring to bed," both in terms of longstanding predispositions and experiences of the past day, will help us guide you more reliably toward the portal to sleep.

• • •

In 1986, Arthur Spielman modeled the course of insomnia in a scheme that remains highly influential, and which serves as the springboard for the present work. Known as the 3P Model of Insomnia, it separates the factors influencing insomnia into three types, differing from each other both conceptually and chronologically. The first P stands for predisposing factors. These are individual characteristics, whether innate or acquired, that set the stage for insomnia. They may not be sufficient to bring about sleep disturbance on their own, but they do bring us closer to a threshold, above which insomnia develops. Examples of the first P include predispositions to depression, anxiety, and hyperarousal.

The second P represents precipitating factors. These are typically external events that add an overlay of stress to predisposing conditions, thereby breaching the insomnia threshold. A precipitating factor is what patients usually have in mind when they say, "This caused my sleep problem." Indeed, it *serves as a trigger*, even though it does not bear full responsibility for the disturbance. Precipitating factors can be traumatic, such the loss of a job, the death of a loved one, or a divorce. However, they can also be subtle enough to escape initial notice, as when the starting time of a job is moved earlier, or when the side effect of a new medication begins to interfere with sleep.

The third *P*, for perpetuating factors, refers to changes in thinking and behavior that arise in response to insomnia, which *maintain* sleep problems once the effects of precipitating factors have receded. For example, after moving to a new city to search for her first job after college, a young woman feels acutely isolated, and develops severe insomnia. She begins oversleeping in the morning, and napping in the afternoon, to compensate for lost sleep. After a few weeks she comes to dread the evening hours, as she anticipates struggles with sleep. She also takes to keeping the television in her bedroom on "for company" all night long.

These responses may indeed bring about short-term relief, but they also make it more likely that her insomnia will persist. That is, they are perpetuating factors. By the time the woman seeks treatment, she may be bewildered by why her sleep is still so poor, given that in the interim she has made some new friends, has found satisfying work, and is finally feeling at home.

Sleep clinicians (ourselves included) generally focus our efforts on the third *P*. Both predisposing and precipitating factors tend to be treated as givens, which will more or less require a workaround. Predisposing factors are long-standing, this thinking goes, and often have received prior treatment. If necessary, such treatment can be resumed or modified, typically by another specialist. And as precipitating factors erupt prior to consultation, their damage is done. Situation-specific interventions such as grief counseling or help with a job search may be beneficial; often the mere passage of time can be counted on to bring some degree of healing.

By contrast, perpetuating factors deal directly with the stuff of sleep and sleeplessness—bedtimes and rising times, sleep-related anxieties, compensatory behaviors, dependence on sleep medications, and the like. What's more, early on it was demonstrated that addressing these factors could bring substantial benefit—within a matter of weeks—to people who had suffered from insomnia for years, regardless of what had originally triggered their disturbance! So it should not be surprising that behavioral sleep specialists mainly target perpetuating factors.

As our field has matured, however, more attention is being paid to the relationship between predisposing factors and sleep. What has been found has been surprising—the relationship can be two-way. Depression is a prime example of this new focus. Sleep disturbance was traditionally assumed to be just a symptom of depression, and was expected to resolve once the mood disorder itself was properly treated. But the consensus today is that the relationship between insomnia and depression is *interactive.* They are now understood to be mutually influencing disturbances, and in fact when the two problems appear together, treating the sleep disturbance can alter the course of the depression.

Similarly, the commonsense perception that sleep disturbance must be the consequence of pain, rather than its trigger, has not survived scientific inquiry. It has been known for some time, for example, that experimental awakenings or restrictions of sleep time will lower thresholds for pain. For the past twenty years there has been a fairly solid consensus that, as with sleep and depression, the relationship between sleep and pain is reciprocal.

More recent work has further shifted the balance, with sleep disturbance often seen as exerting the more powerful effects. Large longitudinal studies (which follow a group of subjects over time) and the use of new statistical techniques have established that the presence of insomnia *at baseline*, for example, is associated with a greater likelihood of developing new-onset headache disorder or fibromyalgia in subsequent years. In patients who are already contending with pain, in conditions as diverse as temporomandibular joint disorder, backache, and fibromyalgia, sleep quality has been demonstrated to *predict* pain flare-ups at later times.

You Are Getting Sleepy is very much in keeping with this trend toward greater appreciation of the interactions between predisposing factors and sleep. Our emphasis is not only on *Getting Sleepy*; it is on *You*, and the specific personal characteristics that can hinder *your* progress across the threshold of sleepiness. We also focus on how insomnia then feeds back on the predisposing factors that contributed to its onset in the first place.

Given that people come to sleep poorly in different ways, some chapters of this book will likely prove more useful to you than others. Everyone should start with chapter 1, as it provides a fresh take on the major non-drug treatments for insomnia—namely, how they address the near-universal problem of **Trying Too Hard** to sleep, by instead working to elicit sleepiness at the right time and place. The chapter also offers a bit of the history and thinking behind the development of these treatments. It mentions some key figures, to whose writings you may wish to refer to learn more. Finally, it presents some less well-validated but promising approaches.

The book's next five chapters are organized around tendencies—whether inborn or acquired long ago—that predispose one to insomnia. These include being **Hyper**, revved up when you should be winding down; **Fatigued**, which typically leads to more rest than sleep; **Depressed**, with its predictable disruptions of sleep architecture; **Anxious**, unable to let go of your worries and drift off; and finally, **Out of Sync** in the timing of your sleep, with personal obligations or societal norms.

You are invited to recognize features in each presentation that match your own leanings. You may spot yourself closely rendered in one particular chapter. Alternatively, you may find that you harbor your own custom blend of predisposing factors, which incline you to insomnia two or three times over. Regardless of how you make your way through these middle sections, all of you will probably want to reconvene at the final chapter on being **Dependent on Medication**, an issue that may loom large for you at present, or is at least potentially of concern.

A focus on factors that predispose you to insomnia can seem a bit unfair, as these tendencies are so deep-rooted. There is only so much you can do about their presence in your life. We encourage you to take heart nonetheless. We have combed through the research literature and surveyed current clinical practice to sort out especially pertinent treatment recommendations, and will take pains to explain why you should give them your full consideration.

Our aim is to speak almost as if we were sitting together at the close of a consultation. We will detail changes you can make to your daily routines to prepare the way for better sleep. We will specify ways in which you can best apply standard cognitive behavioral treatments. And we will introduce new interventions that would seem especially promising for you. We are confident that, taken as a whole, our approach is effective in treating insomnia, *in people like you.*

CHAPTER ONE

———

You are **Trying Too Hard** to Sleep: Aiming for **Sleepiness** Instead

There has never been a shortage of advice regarding how best to sleep. Normal sleepers have their share of "bad nights," while even the most severe insomniacs fall asleep successfully on occasion. So it is not surprising that we should all take stock of our experience, trying to figure out what helps sleep and what gets in its way. The insomnia literature was crowdsourced early on, containing contributions from herbalists, poets, athletes, philosophers, celebrities, physicians, and more than a few hardened insomniacs who somehow found their way back into sleep's good graces. Conspicuously absent from this roll call are the particularly good snoozers, who, in a telling omission, generally do not give sleep much thought.

This plethora of insomnia advice manages to fit neatly into just two categories. The first includes things we can do to or for ourselves: we can count sheep, drink valerian tea, relax our muscles, take sleeping pills, breathe deeply, work out at the gym, try magnesium, practice meditation, see a sleep specialist, and more. The second category includes things we can do to or for our sleeping environment: we can buy a new mattress, stream a soundtrack of rainfall, set out a lavender scent, turn the thermostat down, install blackout curtains, turn the clock out of sight, and so on.

The common thread running through all these suggestions is that there are things *you can do* to get better sleep. Reframed for our information-rich age, there are things *you should know to do*. An early home sleep monitor aimed at consumers, known as the Zeo, emphasized this viewpoint in its advertising slogan, "The More You Know, the Better You Sleep." As sleep clinicians we certainly believe that there *are* things you can do and things you should know to promote better sleep, but we see the situation as slightly more complicated.

In our opinion, Zeo's tagline left out the crucial last step, which is that after you've prepared a comfortable bed in a cool, dark, quiet room, after you've refrained from consuming alcoholic or caffeinated beverages too late in the day—yes, even after you've learned all about the workings of the homeostatic sleep drive and the circadian clock, perhaps from our book *The Insomnia Answer*—you have to *stop doing, stop knowing,* and in short, *stop trying* to sleep. Otherwise you are likely to be awake for a long time. To return to our surfer analogy, you can't go chasing waves, whether they arise from the depths of the ocean or the depths of your brain.

As we observed in our introduction, the standard non-drug treatments for insomnia that coalesced over the last several decades into what is known as Cognitive Behavioral Therapy for Insomnia, or CBT-I, have been covered in several monographs. These include Peter Hauri and Shirley Linde's *No More Sleepless Nights*, Gregg Jacobs's *Say Goodnight to Insomnia*, Colleen Carney and Rachel Manber's *Quiet Your Mind and Get to Sleep*, and Jack Edinger and Colleen Carney's workbook *Overcoming Insomnia*, as well as our own book. Assuming you have been dealing with insomnia for years, they are probably familiar by now.

CBT-I treatments can seem a motley assortment. This is partly because of the differing theoretical orientations of their originators, but also because sleep is so multifaceted. Approaches that emphasize mind, body, and environment all can help. Given all this divergence, it is instructive to revisit the traditional components of CBT-I (as well as some other approaches, both old and new) this time in relation to the single core problem we have been discussing—that of *trying too hard to sleep*.

Before we do, it would be instructive to get a gauge on how much effort characterizes *your* approach to sleep. Colin Espie and his colleagues have developed a model of insomnia in which the effort to sleep plays a prominent role. In connection with this work, they have constructed a simple scale that measures this effort, the Glasgow Sleep Effort Scale. Take a moment to rate these seven statements:

Glasgow Sleep Effort Scale

The following seven statements relate to your nighttime sleep pattern in the past week. Please indicate by circling one response how true each statement is for you.

1   I put too much effort into sleeping when it should come naturally.

   Very much   To some extent   Not at all

2   I feel I should be able to control my sleep.

   Very much   To some extent   Not at all

3   I put off going to bed at night for fear of not being able to sleep.

   Very much   To some extent   Not at all

4   I worry about not sleeping if I cannot sleep.

   Very much   To some extent   Not at all

5   I am no good at sleeping.

   Very much   To some extent   Not at all

6   I get anxious about sleeping before I go to bed.

   Very much   To some extent   Not at all

7   I worry about the consequences of not sleeping.

   Very much   To some extent   Not at all

Niall M. Broomfield and Colin A. Espie. 2005. "Towards a Valid, Reliable Measure of Sleep Effort." *Journal of Sleep Research* 14 (4): 401–407. doi:10.1111/j.1365-2869.2005.00481. Used by permission.

Score 0 points for questions to which you responded "not at all," 1 point for questions answered "to some extent," and 2 points when you agreed "very much." Then add all the points up. In one validation study, the average score for people with insomnia was about 7 points, whereas the average for good sleepers was just slightly over 1 point. In other words, good sleepers responded "not at all" to nearly every question!

Clearly, too much effort to sleep, as well as too many concerns about being unable to sleep, differentiate good and poor sleepers. However, unlike the predisposing factors for insomnia highlighted in coming chapters, these attitudes and behaviors are *reinforced nightly*. They are not coded in your genes, nor have they roots in long-ago trauma. You can just as well learn to approach sleep, and sleeplessness, another way. Cognitive behavioral treatments for insomnia will show you how.

SLEEP HYGIENE RECOMMENDATIONS

A straightforward list of things you can do to sleep better, originally more a distillation of clinical experience but increasingly buttressed by scientifically vetted knowledge, has been collected in the form of "sleep hygiene" guidelines, a term coined by Peter Hauri in 1977. There are various sleep hygiene formulations, but they all cover similar bases, such as:

1. Do not spend too much time in bed. Avoid

napping, and get up at the same time every morning.

2. Sleep in a comfortable bed, in a dark, quiet room that is neither too warm nor too cool.

3. Cut down on caffeinated beverages, and avoid them altogether beyond midafternoon.

4. Refrain from consuming alcohol after dinner.

5. Do not smoke cigarettes in the evening, nor when unable to sleep at night.

6. Do not consume a heavy meal or too much liquid of any type before bedtime. A light snack, however, can be helpful.

7. Get regular exercise, but not too close to bedtime.

8. Wind down during a "buffer period" of an hour or so before bed. Get off your phone, turn off your computer, and don't watch the nightly news or other potentially distressing or overly stimulating shows. Engage in relaxing activity such as reading or listening to music instead.

There is a lot of common sense and potential benefit packed into this compact list. Nonetheless, sleep hygiene recommendations tend to be discounted by poor sleepers. Perhaps it's because they are *too* straightforward and seem to offer nothing new. We can almost guarantee that as we review sleep hygiene recommendations with our patients they will be brushed aside as having been tried before without success. "It didn't make any difference whether I drank coffee or not," we will hear. "Sometimes I will nap and sleep just fine later on, other times I won't nap and still have awful sleep." The message patients convey is that, however it may be for others, their sleep is uniquely erratic. It doesn't respond to commonsense approaches—if it did, they wouldn't be consulting with us!

In a way, doctors tend to give short shrift to sleep hygiene as well. Here, the issue is not one of disbelief but rather of dispatch. Healthcare providers are always pressed for time, and sleep hygiene certainly seems tailor-made for a handout. The intent may be to provide a summary of useful recommendations, and a memory jog when the patient is at home. But if not personalized at least to a modest degree, a printed list of sleep hygiene rules may well be perceived as chiding—"If you would only behave more reasonably, you wouldn't have this sleep problem!"

Dr. Hauri was the first to emphasize that when it comes to sleep, treatment recommendations cannot be reduced to a brochure. It takes clinical judgment to recognize the contributions of individual differences, and make adjustments accordingly. A deep-breathing exercise that one person finds relaxing, for example, can make another person antsy or even trigger panic. Most people would feel too flushed after a hot bath to sleep, while some would find it a soothing prelude. And even when an appropriate behavioral change has been put in place, its benefits may not be immediately apparent due to the night-to-night variability in sleep. It may require a few weeks rather than a few nights to decide whether a particular recommendation is helpful.

We see the elements of sleep hygiene as setting the stage for better sleep. They occasionally lead to remission of chronic insomnia, but usually more focused interventions are required. Our experience is reflected in the consensus paper formulated by the American Academy of Sleep Medicine, titled "Practice Parameters for the Nonpharmacologic Treatment of Chronic Insomnia." In this paper sleep hygiene is seen as a useful adjunct rather than as a standalone treatment for insomnia.

Most (but not all) sleep hygiene recommendations may be understood as *efforts you can make toward better sleep*. It is instructive to consider that the other major components of CBT-I—stimulus control instructions, sleep restriction therapy, and cognitive therapy—despite drawing upon a wide range of theoretical constructs, all at one point or another induce poor sleepers to *stop trying so hard to sleep*. What's more, these CBT-I components provide practical means of accomplishing this tricky assignment. We believe this to be a less heralded but critical ingredient of their success.

STIMULUS CONTROL INSTRUCTIONS

1. Go to bed only when sleepy.
2. If you are not asleep within about twenty minutes, get out of bed and read, listen to quiet music, or just relax in a chair.
3. Don't go back to bed until you are feeling sleepy. If you do go back to bed and have not fallen asleep in about twenty minutes, repeat number 2.
4. Use the bed only for sleep or sex.

5. Wake up at the same time every morning.
6. Don't nap.

Stimulus control instructions were first presented by Richard Bootzin in 1972 to a meeting of the American Psychological Association, and grew to become the most extensively validated treatment for chronic insomnia. It is based on narrowing or "controlling" the responses associated with the particular stimulus of climbing into bed, so that this action is more likely to elicit sleep rather than a host of counterproductive responses such as arousal, tossing and turning, mind racing, and frustration. Many of you reading this book have probably tried stimulus control, and you may be somewhat skeptical about its effectiveness, again at least insofar as you are concerned. We invite you to reconsider your position, keeping in mind two main points of our thesis that at first may seem in opposition—(a) the importance of being sleepy, but also of (b) not trying too hard to sleep. Let's review what the treatment, in a typical formulation, asks of you:

1. Go to bed only when sleepy.

There is much that is deceptively simple about stimulus control, starting with this first directive. More than forty years ago, Dr. Bootzin had already recognized that people in general, and poor sleepers in particular, cannot be counted on to go to bed only when sleepy. As you will learn in coming chapters, they may retire to bed for all sorts of reasons: they're fatigued, the clock says it is "bedtime," they have to get an early start tomorrow, their favorite show is over, their bed partner is turning in, or their feet hurt, to name a few. Whatever the prompt, they are not really *sleepy*. Going to bed for any other reason is a setup for insomnia.

2. If you are not asleep within about twenty minutes, get out of bed and read, listen to quiet music, or just relax in a chair.

This is where you may have given up on stimulus control instructions in the past. Even though you hardly associate your bed and bedroom with warm and fuzzy feelings, staying in bed still feels preferable to sitting up all alone in the middle of the night. You may argue that leaving the bed to read guarantees you won't be slumbering anytime soon. What if this was going to be one of those lucky nights when you would have gotten back to sleep? Or you may counter that moving out of bed and turning on a light to read wakes you up completely.

Our response is that you will definitely lose some *bedtime* by following this instruction, but really not much *sleep*. After all, stimulus control should not be deployed if you are already in a halfway state, on the verge of drifting off. There is no timer set to rouse you out of bed at that point just because twenty minutes have passed. Rather, it is *your own awareness* of time passing, your own growing frustration, that strikes the alarm. Honestly, in your experience, if you have already been lying awake for twenty minutes, growing antsier rather than calmer by the minute, how often are you sleeping a short while later? Think of stimulus control as a kind of "reboot" when things are going haywire. Sometimes it's just better to start over.

At times you may indeed become less sleepy by leaving the bed. You can guard against such arousal by preparing a comfy chair with a throw blanket beforehand. On a side table place a small reading light with an amber or soft pink bulb, some books or magazines, or perhaps headphones and soothing music. You don't want to fall back asleep in the chair, but neither do you want to read for an hour. While your stay should last somewhere around twenty minutes, in our practice we emphasize the concept of *readiness for sleep* inherent in stimulus control, and try to get patients away from a stopwatch mentality. The brief sacrifice of bedtime that this treatment entails yields a key benefit, namely that when you are reading or listening in a chair, *you are no longer trying to sleep*. This leads to the third instruction:

3. Don't go back to bed until you are feeling sleepy. If you do go back to bed and have not fallen asleep in about twenty minutes, repeat number 2.

In following this advice you may occasionally find yourself bouncing between the bed and chair. Again, it's only fair to compare this possibility against the odds that by remaining in bed you'll be awake for hours. A vicious cycle is easily established, with sleepiness giving way to hyperarousal, as the realization that you are not able to sleep is declared an "emergency" in its own right. This pretty much guarantees that you will stay awake to deal with the problem! Breaking this cycle through stimulus control—even if you occasionally make a false start or two—is more likely to unmask latent sleepiness that would have been lost amid all your tossing and turning.

4. Use the bed only for sleep or sex.

This straightforward instruction aims to narrow the associations your bed will elicit. When stimulus control was developed, the time-honored activities of reading and eating in bed had already been joined by watching television and making calls from nightstand phones. We've only become more engaged and connected in bed since, first through laptops and now smartphones. At this point the bed is more command post than refuge. We're on call from work, swapping photos and tweets with friends, pinged by algorithms hawking stock tips, and competing with online gamers on the other side of the world.

The only old-fashioned things in this picture are your neurons, which have not had a chance to evolve over the past fifteen years or so to match this new standard of responsiveness. They still get too excited by random alerts in the middle of the night, and many of them take a long time to calm down even after others have determined that the message wasn't that important in the first place. If you truly wish to sleep well, you must safeguard your bedroom against *all* break-ins, including those of the high-tech variety.

5. Wake up at the same time every morning.

Much research has confirmed the importance of setting or "entraining" the circadian clock by getting light exposure at the same time every morning. For those of you who have trouble falling asleep, this one simple step is probably the single most important change you can make. We'll have a lot more to say about it in a later chapter. Here we focus on an aspect that often gets in the way of compliance: most everyone is loath to forego the chance to "catch up" on sleep after a fitful night. Mind and body, at odds over so much in life, are united when it comes to oversleeping. Your brain will come up with all sorts of reasons for staying in bed even if you did manage to set an alarm, while your muscles will resist any stray impulse to move.

We know how hard it is, but we urge you to follow this directive the best you can. Waking at the same time every day (in our practice we allow a rising time up to one hour later on weekends, if necessary, to maintain morale) taps into the two fundamental mechanisms regulating sleep—the homeostatic sleep drive, which strengthens when sleep is cut short, and, as noted above, the circadian clock. Starting your day on schedule will also demonstrate that you can get by despite poor sleep. You'll see yourself rally when circumstances warrant decisive action, and be able to muddle through when nothing critical is going on. We're the first to espouse the importance of sleep, but paradoxically, you'll get more of it overall if you downplay the need to get an optimal amount every night.

6. Don't nap.

This is another tried-and-true recommendation more recently given theoretical underpinnings. We understand that many people (as well as some entire cultures) do well with an afternoon nap, and considerable research has accumulated regarding the restorative effects of naps when nocturnal sleep is restricted by external demands. For example, periods of wakefulness lasting thirty-six hours or longer are sometimes required during public safety emergencies or military operations. Academic studies simulating these conditions have demonstrated that relatively brief naps, on the order of one to two hours, can yield major improvements in performance during intervening stretches of prolonged wakefulness.

However, in everyday life, for those of you who are already having a hard time sleeping at night, it is counterproductive to expend your sleep drive during the day. It is also detrimental to "flatten" the waking portion of your sleep/wake cycle with periods of bedrest, whether or not you doze. This is especially true for those who are aiming for a "full night" of sleep *plus* a nap, in the belief that you're at your well-rested best under those conditions. There are some naturally "long sleepers" who can pull off this feat, but since you are reading this book you are probably not among them!

SLEEP RESTRICTION THERAPY

It is an amusing sidelight of CBT-I that most of its key components have names that range from the problematic to the unfortunate. Dr. Hauri was often asked about the turn-of-the-[previous]-century connotations of "sleep *hygiene*," and he used to answer with his unique straight-faced smile that he didn't like it either, while challenging his interlocutor to come up with something better. After several decades of prominence as a treatment, the meaning of "Stimulus Control Instructions" remains quizzical to nearly all general physicians, and more than a few sleep specialists, let alone their patients. One of us may have continued this trend when, in the interest of full disclosure, he settled on Sleep Restriction Therapy (SRT) as the name of his new behavioral treatment for insomnia. Ever since, insomnia patients have approached the treatment with a mixture of apprehension and incredulity that sometimes requires considerable clinical finesse to allay.

That apprehension may be justified, by not only the name but the substance of treatment. After all, SRT originated in observations gleaned from research on the effects of partial sleep deprivation, a scientific literature that had burgeoned in the 1960s and 1970s. It was learned from these studies that when sleep is repeatedly cut short by several hours, its internal "architecture" changes in predictable ways. For starters, people fall asleep more quickly when given the chance—by definition, *they get sleepier*.

Bedtime is also used more "efficiently" to accumulate the most sleep possible under the circumstances, squeezing out wakefulness. Relatively more time is spent in the

Into bed

Alcohol

Medication
1 = Benadryl, 50mg

Asleep

Out of bed

Caffeine

A

1

C

6 7 8 9 10 11 Mid 1 2 3 4 5 6 7 8 9 10 11 Noon 1 2 3 4 5 6

Morning's Date	Time to Fall Asleep	Amount of Sleep	Sleep Quality 1 Lo–10 Hi
Mon 12/10	100 min	5 hours	3

Medication 1 _____ mg   Medication 2 _____ mg

deepest, most restorative stage of non-rapid eye movement (NREM) sleep, with its high threshold for arousal, and less time is spent in the lighter NREM stages. Rapid eye movement (REM) sleep, the stage associated with vivid dreaming, is also curtailed. This is so because most of a given night's REM sleep takes place in the final hours of sleep, the very hours that are lost under a restricted regimen.

The essence of SRT involves closely matching the time you are allowed in bed to the time you estimate you spend sleeping, as deduced from sleep logs such as the one provided here. For example, say you kept a two-week log showing that you spent an average of 8.5 hours in bed, but you estimated sleep to average only 6 hours. Your "sleep efficiency" (time estimated asleep/time spent in bed) is 6/8.5, or just over 70 percent. By comparison, during a good night of sleep this figure would be closer to 90 percent.

In this example, under SRT you would be assigned an initial time in bed of six hours. (Note that we usually provide a minimum duration of five hours, so that even if you estimated only three-and-a-half hours of sleep, we would still assign you five hours in bed.) Where do we cut back on bedtime? Since many people with chronic sleep difficulties go to bed early, in an unsuccessful attempt to capture more sleep, we usually end up assigning a later time to get into bed. However, we also take into account when the logs indicate sleep to be most likely. So, if your logs showed consistent, prolonged awakenings toward morning, we would move your rising time earlier to reduce time in bed.

Over the subsequent week, the major reduction in time in bed imposed by SRT is typically accompanied by only a modest reduction in estimated sleep time. This results in much-improved sleep efficiency. For example, your next log might show an average of five-and-a-half hours of sleep during your assigned six hours in bed, yielding a very good sleep efficiency of just below 92 percent. Thereafter, the amount of time you spent in bed would be adjusted according to how efficiently you filled that time with sleep.

In the original formulation of SRT, time in bed was extended by fifteen minutes if sleep efficiency calculated from the previous week's log was over 90 percent, while time in bed was reduced by fifteen minutes if the sleep efficiency was below 85 percent. If it fell between these two cutoffs, no change was made for the coming week. We and other sleep clinicians subsequently proposed modifications of this scheme—for example, lowering the threshold for extending time in bed to 85 percent for the elderly.

In current practice we often employ a simplified SRT strategy. It involves just one initial restriction, to match the average sleep time on baseline logs. Subsequently, allotted time in bed either increases or holds steady, avoiding the demoralization that further tightening of time in bed can prompt. The decision to increase or hold steady depends on how much total wakefulness (time spent waiting to fall asleep *plus* wakefulness after sleep onset) is estimated to occur nightly. This threshold varies between patients; it is typically forty-five minutes.

If, averaged across the past week, wakefulness equals or exceeds the threshold, the initial restricted schedule is maintained. If wakefulness dips below the threshold, fifteen minutes are added to time in bed. The extra time is added to one side of the night or the other in a consistent fashion. This process is repeated weekly, to find the longest time in bed that can typically be filled with sleep while still keeping wakefulness to an agreed-upon minimum.

Sleep Restriction Therapy (Simplified Version)

1. Fill out a one-week baseline sleep log. Make sure that your log records **time into bed**, **time out of bed**, and estimated **sleep time**. From the log, calculate **time spent in bed** (**time into bed** until **time out of bed**) each night.

2. Add up **time spent in bed** across the week and divide by seven to yield **average time spent in bed**.

3. Add up **sleep time** across the week and divide by seven to yield **average sleep time**.

4. Subtract **average sleep time** from **average time in bed** to yield **average wake time**.

5. During the first week of treatment, set your **restricted time in bed** equal to the **average sleep time** calculated from your baseline log. If **average sleep time** is less than five hours, allow yourself five hours in bed. Continue to keep your sleep log.

6. At the end of the next week, if **average wake time** is less than forty-five minutes, add fifteen minutes to your **restricted time in bed**. You may add it to the beginning or end of the night, but be consistent. If **average wake time** is greater than or equal to forty-five minutes, remain on your current schedule.

7. Repeat step 6 until you arrive at the longest **restricted time in bed** that consistently yields an average wake time of about forty-five minutes.

SRT clearly fits the paradigm we have been discussing, that of not trying so hard to sleep. With its late bedtimes, early rising times, and prohibition against "catching up" on sleep, the treatment is more aptly characterized as requiring effort to stay awake! People who have long struggled with insomnia are often incredulous that they should forego the possibility of sleep. However, there is method to this madness: forcing yourself to stay awake may be difficult, but it *can be done*, and that in turn will help you sleep. By contrast, you simply cannot force yourself asleep.

By holding out for that occasional "great night," you have been kept in thrall to a losing proposition, the way random payoffs keep gamblers at slot machines as their money drains away. Under SRT there are no more jackpots. Your sleep will even out—it will not be great, but it will not be terrible either. Shorter times in bed with less wakefulness also means that there will be less time for intrusive thoughts, less time for mind racing. Ultimately we want your sleep to become predictable and boring. Just as good sleepers don't give much thought to how they will sleep on a given night, sleep should eventually become a no-brainer for you as well.

COGNITIVE THERAPY FOR INSOMNIA

You may be thinking at this point, "A no-brainer—fat chance of that!" Right now sleep is about *all* you think about. You are reminded of it as you try to maintain focus on work assignments, as you muster the energy to tackle household chores. By the time dusk falls, the anticipation of yet another sleepless night is bound to be front and center in your thoughts.

Plus, you have long-term concerns. Is your brain somehow broken? Will mental lapses be cited on your next performance review? How can your health hold up if you go practically sleepless night after night? It's hard enough to trudge through life without enough sleep; can you really be expected to do so without worrying about it?

We agree that your sleep is a cause for concern—that's why, after all, you are reading this book. However, there is a big range between concern and full-blown panic. Are you among the many poor sleepers who, faced with the apparent breakdown of such a basic life function, have developed catastrophic reactions? Are you convinced that you will never sleep well again? Are you ever on the lookout for damage done, and quick to attribute any and all problems to your sleeplessness? Such reactions not only go beyond what the evidence justifies, they also stoke cognitive hyper-arousal, which, as you'll read in the next chapter, will make sleep even harder to come by.

Charles Morin and his colleagues have done much work identifying maladaptive cognitive reactions to the experience of chronically poor sleep. These have been collated into the Dysfunctional Beliefs and Attitudes about

Sleep (DBAS) scale, originally a set of thirty statements, subsequently winnowed down to sixteen. It may prove helpful to get a reflection of *your* beliefs and attitudes about sleep, as a starting point for determining which ones you might wish to challenge, by completing the scale yourself.

Beliefs about Sleep

Several statements reflecting people's beliefs and attitudes about sleep are listed below. Please indicate (by *circling the number*) to what extent you personally agree or disagree with each statement. There is no right or wrong answer. For each statement, circle a number that best reflects your personal experience. Consider the whole scale, rather than only the extremes of the continuum.

1   **I need eight hours of sleep to feel refreshed and function well during the day.**

Strongly Disagree 0 1 2 3 4 5 6 7 8 9 10 Strongly Agree

2   **When I do not get a proper amount of sleep on a given night, I need to catch up on the next day by napping or on the next night by sleeping longer.**

Strongly Disagree 0 1 2 3 4 5 6 7 8 9 10 Strongly Agree

3   **I am concerned that chronic insomnia may have serious consequences for my physical health.**

Strongly Disagree 0 1 2 3 4 5 6 7 8 9 10 Strongly Agree

4   **I am worried that I may lose control over my ability to sleep.**

Strongly Disagree 0 1 2 3 4 5 6 7 8 9 10 Strongly Agree

5   After a poor night's sleep, I know that it will interfere with my daily activities on the next day.

Strongly Disagree 0 1 2 3 4 5 6 7 8 9 10 Strongly Agree

6   In order to be alert and function well during the day, I am better off taking a sleeping pill rather than having a poor night's sleep.

Strongly Disagree 0 1 2 3 4 5 6 7 8 9 10 Strongly Agree

7   When I feel irritable, depressed, or anxious during the day, it is mostly because I did not sleep well the night before.

Strongly Disagree 0 1 2 3 4 5 6 7 8 9 10 Strongly Agree

8   When I sleep poorly on one night, I know that it will disturb my sleep schedule for the whole week.

Strongly Disagree 0 1 2 3 4 5 6 7 8 9 10 Strongly Agree

9   Without an adequate night's sleep, I can hardly function the next day.

Strongly Disagree 0 1 2 3 4 5 6 7 8 9 10 Strongly Agree

10   I can't ever predict whether I will have a good or poor night's sleep.

Strongly Disagree 0 1 2 3 4 5 6 7 8 9 10 Strongly Agree

11   I have little ability to manage the negative consequences of disturbed sleep.

Strongly Disagree 0 1 2 3 4 5 6 7 8 9 10 Strongly Agree

12 When I feel tired, have no energy, or just seem not to function well during the day, it is generally because I did not sleep well the night before.

Strongly Disagree 0 1 2 3 4 5 6 7 8 9 10 Strongly Agree

13 I believe that insomnia is essentially a result of a chemical imbalance.

Strongly Disagree 0 1 2 3 4 5 6 7 8 9 10 Strongly Agree

14 I feel that insomnia is ruining my ability to enjoy life and prevents me from doing what I want.

Strongly Disagree 0 1 2 3 4 5 6 7 8 9 10 Strongly Agree

15 Medication is probably the only solution to sleeplessness.

Strongly Disagree 0 1 2 3 4 5 6 7 8 9 10 Strongly Agree

16 I avoid or cancel obligations (social, family, occupational) after a poor night's sleep.

Strongly Disagree 0 1 2 3 4 5 6 7 8 9 10 Strongly Agree

Charles M. Morin, Annie Vallières, and Hans Ivers. 2007. "Dysfunctional Beliefs and Attitudes about Sleep (DBAS): Validation of a Brief Version (DBAS-16)." *Sleep* 30 (11): 1547–1554. Used by permission.

How many of these beliefs and attitudes did you tend to agree with? While they differentiate both statistically and clinically between good and poor sleepers, what is especially important for you is that they can be *changed*, whether through self-reflection or with the aid of cognitive therapy. And if you can put your mind at ease *about* sleep, you'll be much more able to ease your mind *into* sleep.

In the more than twenty years since the initial publication of the DBAS, numerous insomnia-related research findings have been picked up by mainstream media to cause many of you deep concern. These include growing evidence that some chronic sleep and circadian rhythm disorders are *indeed* linked to a broad array of health risks—in cardiovascular, gastrointestinal, endocrine, cognitive, metabolic, and other realms. Health issues can crop up when sleep is mistimed, habitually broken by arousals, or of limited duration—problems you are likely quite familiar with. How can we possibly allay these and other concerns, when they are becoming more and more evidence-based?

Before this literature became established we could at least reassure our patients that, since the "deepest" (NREM stage 3, or slow-wave) sleep appeared in the first hours of sleep, a full quotient might still be accumulated in an otherwise miserable half night. However, the preservation of deep sleep is evidently not sufficient to ward off the health consequences of missing out on too much of the lighter stages. (Some of you may be under the impression that REM sleep is the deepest or most restorative stage. Actually, the brain in REM is quite activated, producing dreams, consolidating memories, and extracting the gist of recent emotional and intellectual experiences. Given all this activity, it's perhaps not surprising that the EEG of REM sleep is sometimes difficult to differentiate from wakefulness! In one regard, however, REM sleep is deep: it's the most difficult stage from which to arouse a sleeper, as attempts to do so are often incorporated into ongoing dream imagery. REM sleep's combination of an awake-like EEG and a high threshold for arousal has led the stage to be called "paradoxical sleep.")

Similarly, we can no longer count on the likelihood that you are probably getting somewhat more sleep than you subjectively estimate. After all, much of the research on habitual sleep length and either specific health problems or overall life expectancy has been based on survey data, which *also* relies on subjective estimates of sleep.

We believe it best in the long run to just go ahead and acknowledge that sleep is an integral part of living, and that future research will likely bind it ever more closely to virtually all aspects of waking life. You can take solace in knowing that there is still much to sort out with regard to sleep and health, and plenty of anomalies—like Thomas Edison, who lived to eighty-four and was nothing if not productive on his four hours of sleep—left to explain. In the meantime, there are many other dysfunctional thoughts you can target!

For starters, we are confident that you can be a *better* sleeper than you are now, and thereby lower whatever risk you face. It is the rare person who has managed to avoid *every* maladaptive response to chronic insomnia. Each represents an opportunity for improvement. Take a personal inventory, and see if your history of poor sleep has not indeed fanned anxieties over your prospects for sleep tonight, or the thought of struggling through tomorrow. Check whether the lack of sleep has prompted you to extend your time in bed in the hopes of catching more. Do you now tend to "crash" into sleep rather than winding down properly? Have you become dependent upon sedating or hypnotic medication? The list goes on. So there is in fact much to improve, starting with the overarching dysfunctional thought that *your insomnia cannot be helped.*

Next, you might reexamine your belief that *everything hinges on sleep.* It does not detract a bit from the accruing literature on the links between sleep disturbance and insulin resistance, for example, to allow that other interventions, such as switching away from sugary drinks or increasing physical activity, may still be helpful in warding off type II diabetes. It is a fallacy to assume that the particular risk factor especially pertinent to you is the only one that can make a difference.

Finally, what about coming up with a more realistic appraisal of the risks you face? Do you really think that, just because researchers are finally confirming long-assumed connections between sleep and well-being, *you are suddenly at increased risk*? That you and your fellow insomniacs will be dropping like flies now that clinical understanding has advanced? Just a little reflection should convince you that insomnia is an age-old scourge; its consequences were long ago "baked into" our collective experience. No, we would argue that even for you, discoveries of specific health risks associated with poor sleep represent *a net benefit.* While they have not in themselves increased your risk one iota, they may well lead to specific precautionary recommendations that will improve your health in the long run.

WHILE YOU ARE AWAKE

We have reviewed four core components of CBT-I—sleep hygiene, stimulus control instructions, sleep restriction therapy, and cognitive therapy for insomnia—from the perspective of how each addresses the problem of trying too hard to sleep. While originating from quite different perspectives, they all soothe this urgency by suggesting changes in behaviors and thoughts surrounding the experience of sleeplessness.

There are several other approaches that, rather than targeting better sleep, in essence aim for better *wakefulness*—in the sense of being calmer, more composed, and more present-focused. Although techniques such as progressive relaxation, autogenic training, and mindfulness-based stress reduction were not specifically formulated as insomnia treatments, they have all been employed to improve sleep, often with encouraging results. This is likely because such treatments can quiet both the physiological and cognitive hyperarousal that so readily inhibits sleep.

Progressive Relaxation

Progressive relaxation was introduced by Edmund Jacobson in 1929. Its current form typically involves tensing and then relaxing muscle groups in sequence—either from toes to head or in the opposite direction—with the aim of learning to recognize and appreciate the state of relaxation in these muscles. Before practicing this technique, find a quiet place in which to sit or lie comfortably, wear loose clothing, and remove your shoes.

Within each muscle group, focus on one side of your body and then the other before moving on—e.g., right foot, left foot, right calf, left calf, right thigh, left thigh, and so on. As you inhale, tense the muscles in your targeted group hard for about five seconds, and then, as you exhale, ease those same muscles into a relaxed state for at least fifteen seconds. Attend especially to the sensation of "letting go," of *what it feels like to relax*. The ability to recognize how muscles feel in a relaxed state is a key aspect of this treatment.

Progressive relaxation might be considered limited in its targeting of muscle tension, which is just one manifestation of stress and anxiety. Jacobson's original conception of "neuromuscular hypertension" was significantly broader, encompassing other aspects of what today we would call "physiological hyperarousal" such as an increased heart rate, shallow breathing and restlessness. It does appear to induce a more generalized "relaxation response," to use the term popularized by Herbert Benson nearly fifty years later. Perhaps the most important contribution of Jacobson, from our perspective as insomnia specialists, was his recognition that we do not automatically return to a resting state after the stimulation of work, physical exertion, or even entertainment. We must learn instead to sense our "residual tension," and take active steps to address it, if we wish to be sleepy at bedtime.

Autogenic Training

Autogenic training was popularized by a 1959 book of the same name by two German physicians, Johannes Schultz and Wolfgang Luthe, after having been developed by Schultz nearly thirty years earlier. The method employs a series of self-suggestive statements, e.g., "My right arm is feeling heavier and warmer," to induce feelings of heaviness, warmth, and calm in the limbs, as well as a contrasting coolness in the forehead. In some renditions it also aims for sensations of steadiness, comfort, and calm in the heart rate, respiration, and the stomach. In contrast to the more specific muscle groups targeted by progressive relaxation, limbs are treated as a whole, perhaps first on the right side, then on the left, and then bilaterally.

The effectiveness of autogenic training for the treatment of insomnia is attested to mainly by clinical anecdotes, although there are a few systematic studies extending back to the late 1960s and 1970s that suggest benefit. It might be relegated to the category of relaxation techniques that are in all likelihood good for you, if not particularly specific to insomnia, but for findings in an area of research touched on by another German physician and researcher, Jurgen Aschoff.

In 1958 Aschoff and his colleague Rutger Wever described how temperature in the human body is regulated by transferring heat produced by the brain and internal organs (the "core") to the limbs and extremities (the "shell") and then out to the surrounding environment. Through changes in the path of blood flow and the degree of vascular dilation or constriction, heat carried by the blood is either facilitated on its way out of the body (to cool the "core" in hot environments) or released more sparingly (to stay warm under cold conditions).

Subsequent work has shown that this transfer of heat is intimately connected with your circadian sleep/wake cycle. In the evening, core body heat is transferred to your fingers and toes ("distal" regions, in anatomic parlance). These extremities, because they have a lot of surface area relative to their size and come equipped with special shunts to quickly move blood around their tips, function like little radiators, releasing heat into the environment very efficiently. It is now well established that this "distal warming" (relative to the temperature of the "proximal" trunk covering your internal organs) *predicts the ability to fall asleep quickly.* This makes sense to sleep researchers, since we sleep best when our core temperature is low, and cooling of the brain has long been surmised to be one of the functions of sleep.

A series of studies by Kurt Krauchi and colleagues has clarified the nature of the relationship between heat transfer and sleep, and raised the intriguing possibility of using distal warming to treat insomnia. They found that the transfer of core body heat to the extremities *precedes* sleep onset. It is *not* the result of sleep—merely lying down and relaxing triggers the process. Subsequently, *afferent* signals (signals originating in sensory neurons, here in the fingers and toes, and traveling *toward* the brain centers regulating sleep) confirm that distal warming has occurred. In short, the sensation of warmth in the fingers and toes induces sleepiness.

Understandably, investigators have been busy looking into the effects on sleep of directly warming the hands or feet, whether by traditional means such as gloves or warm socks, or through specially designed warming treatments. It seems plausible that the same neural mechanisms may also be activated by autogenic training, although this remains to be demonstrated.

Mindfulness Meditation

While elements of both progressive relaxation and autogenic training can be traced to ancient Eastern practices, the techniques of mindfulness meditation are explicitly drawn from that tradition. A modern form known as Mindfulness-Based Stress Reduction (MBSR) was developed by Jon Kabat-Zinn in the 1980s and first presented in his book *Full Catastrophe Living* in 1990. Typically imparted in courses spanning about eight weeks, MBSR is now widely used in integrative medicine settings to ameliorate various stress-related disorders, chronic illnesses, and other health problems.

Several groups are researching applications of mindfulness techniques for treating insomnia. Jason Ong and colleagues, for example, have integrated MSBR with elements of traditional CBT-I to form Mindfulness-Based Treatment for Insomnia (MBTI). They are building a case for the effectiveness of this treatment through a series of studies that now range from pilot work to a modest-sized but randomly controlled investigation, published in 2014, in which both the MSBR and MBTI treatments produced substantially greater reductions in presleep hyperarousal and subjectively recorded wakefulness at night, compared to a control group that was self-monitoring sleep using diaries.

Mindfulness—maintaining a nonjudgmental, present-focused awareness, in which self-recrimination for past failings and striving toward future objectives give way to an accepting, inquisitive experience of the moment—is gradually achieved in part through meditation exercises, as well as when opportunities arise for informal application of its precepts. As the practice of mindfulness becomes more established and reflexive, it also becomes very well suited to counter presleep hyperarousal. A brief review of your mental state at bedtime should make clear why this might be so.

Consider the thoughts that typically race around your mind as you lie in the dark each night, and all the anxiety, second-guessing, helplessness, and other distress they kick up: "I hope I didn't make a fool of myself at the presentation today." "What is that strange noise the refrigerator is making?" "Alice seemed so cool this evening." "Will I ever sleep normally again?" "Is all this sleeplessness going to make me sick?"

What if, instead of being strapped to such thoughts like a harnessed racer, propelled into seemingly endless laps around the mental track, you could just step over to the sidelines and observe them? Yes, you would still be able to see a particular notion whirling by as a problem. You could even acknowledge it to be your problem. However, *you wouldn't be hurtling along with it anymore.* Instead, you would now be in position to see it for what it is—just a racing thought, in essence going nowhere. From that vantage point, you might find yourself growing disinterested, and even a bit sleepy. You'll deal with it, the best you can, in the morning.

• • •

The next five chapters address personal characteristics that commonly set the stage for insomnia. As noted in our introduction, it is our experience that several of these factors may be at work, to varying degrees, within a given individual. We are relying on you to recognize which are especially pertinent. Feel free to skip around, based on your personal priorities.

You may also choose to read this book straight through. We have tried our best to minimize repetition, by changing our emphases and tailoring recommendations according to the context of each chapter. You are therefore likely to discover new information about insomnia, and sleep in general, throughout its pages.

Whichever path you take, we recommend reading the last chapter on medication. While some of you may be congenitally prone to drug dependence, in a manner analogous to the other traits discussed, dependence on sleep aids can potentially affect anyone with insomnia. As sleeplessness becomes chronic, anticipatory anxiety over the prospect of yet another poor night develops. When this anxiety is temporarily allayed by pills, it strongly reinforces their continued use.

CHAPTER SUMMARY

- Trying too hard to sleep is counterproductive. Rather than striving for sleep, your objective should be to get sleepy. Sleepiness is the threshold of sleep, as close as you can get to it through your own efforts. You can reliably get sleepy, for example, by learning to disengage your mind from daily concerns, avoiding caffeine late in the day, or restricting time in bed. If you are sleepy at the right time and place, good sleep will come to you.

- Insomnia is a multifaceted problem, and its treatments can seem a motley assortment. We see sleepiness as the final common pathway toward which these treatments converge. For example, stimulus control instructions promote sleepiness by strengthening associations between the bed and sleep, sleep restriction therapy by increasing homeostatic sleep drive, and mindfulness-based techniques by quieting racing or intrusive thoughts.

- In this chapter, we examined how seven treatments promote sleepiness at bedtime. The first four are typical components of what is known as Cognitive Behavioral Therapy for Insomnia, or CBT-I, and are, as that name suggests, expressly concerned with sleep-related behaviors and thoughts:
  - Sleep Hygiene Recommendations
  - Stimulus Control Instructions
  - Sleep Restriction Therapy
  - Cognitive Therapy for Insomnia

- The next three treatments, based on venerable traditions, promote calmer, more balanced waking hours. They indirectly prepare you for sleepiness, and better sleep, at night.

- · Progressive Relaxation
- · Autogenic Training
- · Mindfulness Meditation

- You are predisposed to insomnia by a unique combination of factors; your therapy should be optimized to reflect that mix. Sometimes this will be a matter of emphasizing certain core treatments. At other times, specialized interventions—such as administering bright light treatment or issuing guidelines for resting—may be indicated. In the chapters that follow, we match a number of tailored therapeutic approaches to common predisposing factors for insomnia. Some combination of these strategies will help you find your way to sleep.

CHAPTER TWO

Are You **Too Hyper** to Sleep?

Did you know that a "sleep switch" in the brain has actually been discovered? We're pretty sure this is news to you. After all, there must have been countless times in the past when you longed to locate just such a toggle, or for that matter any other way to turn off your runaway mind. "Switch" is a particularly fitting description of this mechanism, because it seems that one of its purposes is to provide a definitive "click" into either wakefulness or sleep. Otherwise we would be prone to vacillating between the two states like a blinking bulb.

While you were trying to fall asleep last night, you may have deduced a key feature of the sleep switch: it can't be forced. Rather, it flips itself when conditions are right, one of those conditions being *a low level of arousal*. This is very different from being physically exhausted, mentally depleted, or simply done with what you've been doing. So, if you're a waiter who just worked a dinner shift nonstop, prepped for the next day, somehow made it home in one piece, and straggled into bed, you aren't necessarily going to fall asleep. If you're a student who by 3 A.M. finally feels prepared for tomorrow's exam after having reviewed every last note and formula, you may well spend the remaining hours before daybreak staring at the ceiling. Even if you're just having fun—say, a crossword enthusiast partway through a particularly challenging puzzle—once in bed you will probably rummage through unsolved clues rather than sleep.

AROUSAL VS. HYPERAROUSAL

In each of these examples, instead of constituting a wind-down period, nocturnal activities led to *higher* arousal levels—in fact, to a state aptly named *hyperarousal*. Hyperarousal takes two forms—*physiological*, manifest in such bodily changes as a rapid heart rate or increased muscle tension, and *cognitive*, as exemplified by a racing mind. Either type can be quite effective at fending off sleep.

Hyperarousal bears similarities to the "acute stress response" triggered in many animals by an overwhelming threat, often referred to as the "fight or flight" response. It may develop in reaction to specific traumatic events—thereby becoming a core component of posttraumatic stress disorder (PTSD). However, hyperarousal differs from the acute stress response in that it can also build up gradually, in response to accumulated stressors that are not outright emergencies. Finally, it can present as a "trait," a relatively stable personality characteristic, hardwired on a genetic basis rather than being reactive to particular events. Whereas animals cannot sustain a full-fledged fight-or-flight response very long before succumbing to exhaustion, hyperarousal can linger without any definitive action being taken in either the "fight" or the "flight" direction, sometimes to the point of becoming a way of life.

As its name suggests, hyperarousal can be thought of as an exaggerated form of arousal. However, there is a crucial difference. Normal arousal, or what we think of as alertness, follows *a predictable circadian rhythm*. It is the manifestation of the "alerting force" we spoke of in *The Insomnia Answer*. Typically at its lowest in the very early morning, the alerting force gathers strength through the day, to counter a likewise strengthening homeostatic sleep drive and maintain alertness through long hours of wakefulness. The alerting force reaches its peak in the evening. As it rounds that peak and finally begins to weaken at night, the sleep drive gains the upper hand, and we grow sleepy. By contrast, hyperarousal may surge *at any time*, whenever stressful conditions are encountered. Under those stressful conditions it can be quite helpful, at least initially.

HYPERAROUSAL TRIGGERS

If you've just come off a dinner shift, for example, you probably waited on dozens of parties, many arriving in clusters. You had to keep orders straight, work around kitchen bottlenecks, and soothe impatient customers, all the while dashing around tables balancing plates. No doubt you welcomed feeling some extra oomph as you worked. However, that press of activity built up hyperarousal like a head of steam. During the very hours when most people were winding down in anticipation of bedtime, you were in a rush that kept you going until the last dishes were cleared.

By the time you got home it was well past midnight, and plenty of sleep drive had accrued from your extended hours of wakefulness. Your alerting force was definitely waning. You were totally exhausted and headed straight into bed. *So why aren't you sleepy now?*

The answer is hyperarousal, arising from both your physical and mental efforts. Only an hour or two ago it was a saving grace, a genie summoned to help you function during the last hours of your shift. Now it has become an obstruction to sleep. Like a genie, hyperarousal can be difficult to stuff back into its bottle once the task at hand has been fulfilled. By and large it takes us several hours to wind down after intense engagement. By climbing right into bed you've essentially elected to do your winding down there—a venue that is surprisingly unsuited for the task.

You might think that cramming for a test late into the night would trigger cognitive as opposed to physiological hyperarousal, but in fact both outcomes are possible. Your mind is in overdrive, yes, but in addition you may have to contend with the muscle tension, rapid heart rate, shallow breathing, and other physical manifestations of old-fashioned test anxiety. Whether you are a waiter or student (and we know some of you wear both hats!) the problem remains that if you are immersed in work too close to bedtime, sleep may be deferred for hours.

Crossword enthusiasts present a different scenario, in that their late-night activity is not compelled by economic or academic pressure. (We could just as easily substitute here the software engineer who "unwinds" with commando-style video games before turning in, or the teenager who lies in bed texting friends.) No doubt some of your friends can engage in such activities and still fall right off to sleep. Why don't they also make *you* sleepy?

TRAIT HYPERAROUSAL

You remain wide-eyed after your device has powered down in part because of your genes. We all vary with respect to the trait component of hyperarousal: some of us are generally placid and easygoing, while others habitually operate in high gear. We also differ as to how much stimulation is required to trigger a surge of hyperarousal, and how readily we can settle ourselves once the excitement is over.

Anchoring one end of the spectrum are those of you who virtually *never* calm down, who from birth have been a "bundle of energy." In the crib you were up much of the night, often babbling contentedly. The next day you would be hyperactive, yes, but often surprisingly free of crankiness. Brief stints of sleep characterized your school years, and this pattern has persisted into adulthood. Today you are free to turn to your phone to fill in the gaps at night—but as we have seen, this is not likely to hasten sleep. In earlier clinical parlance, you might have been diagnosed with *idiopathic insomnia*, which meant in essence that you were unable to sleep for no clear reason, perhaps other than who you were. Nowadays the role of trait hyperarousal, in what is termed your *primary insomnia*, is being elucidated on a neuronal and genetic level.

By day those of you with inborn hyperarousal tend to be very alert, frenetic, multitracking souls. In the right kind of environment you can put these qualities to good use. You shine, for instance, when it comes to productivity and attention to detail. A reckoning, however, arrives each evening. You are just not equipped with the brakes to counter all that energy, so you end up coasting a very long while into the night before finally coming to a halt.

POSTTRAUMATIC HYPERAROUSAL

Hyperarousal can look quite different in those who acquire it after birth. Those of you contending with PTSD, for example, were probably shaking your heads in disbelief at the peppy, productive picture described above. Your hyperarousal is altogether different: it is alloyed with irritability, hypervigilance, and anxiety. By day you are too jumpy, and have too much difficulty concentrating and staying on task to get much of anything done. While you certainly have plenty of difficulty sleeping now, the course of your insomnia has been different. You remember a time when you could indeed apply the brakes and ease yourself into sleep. It's just that now *you won't let yourself*, given what you've been through. There are too many dangers prowling outside, too many threats lurking in memory, to allow you to stand down and shut both eyes at once.

We will be offering specific recommendations for contending with the hyperarousal of PTSD later in this chapter. First, let's turn to those of you who are unable to calm yourself down either because of shift work or because of choices you make nightly that stoke hyperarousal in the hours before bedtime. Our twofold prescription in your case is easy to state, but not so easy to put into practice: you will need to change how you spend your evening hours, and you will need to change when you turn out the lights.

GETTING SLEEPY AFTER THE EVENING SHIFT

If you work an evening shift and have difficulty falling asleep, you would almost certainly benefit from a *later* bedtime. The biological clocks of most day shift workers are timed to sustain alertness in the early evening while still facilitating sleep before midnight. However, given your active evening hours, your underlying circadian rhythms are likely delayed. Add to this circadian delay the hyperarousal generated by work demands, and the result is that you are in no way sleepy, in the sense of being ready for sleep, when you arrive home. If you go to bed at that time, you will just toss and turn. Instead, you should maintain a wind-down period outside of the bedroom of at least one hour, even if that means a bedtime of 1 A.M. or later.

We can hear the groans. Many of you have children who must be up early for school, and all of you have a list of errands to complete in the shortened day before your next shift begins. You must get to bed right away if you're to make it through. Still, how much sleep are you really getting during that first hour or so in bed? How often must you resort to using a sleep aid, and how successful are those pills against all your fitfulness?

When working with patients directly we are able to formulate treatment plans together, taking the exigencies of their daily lives into account. For you, we do not know if the workaround will involve a partner who lets you sleep later by getting the kids off to school, a nap before work, a tweak to your work hours, or some other fix. All we can say is that if hyperarousal resulting from evening shift work is hindering your sleep, you should not be turning in anywhere near the same time as those who finish up work at 5 P.M.

STAYING SLEEPY IS THE PROBLEM AFTER A NIGHT SHIFT

Those of you working the night shift likely noticed a discrepancy between what you've been reading and your own experience: By the time you straggle home after your shift ends at 7 or 8 A.M., you often *are* ready for sleep, and can drop off quickly. The problem is that you can't stay asleep for more than four or five hours into the day.

The reason you can readily fall asleep in the morning (and also the reason why you wake up too early) has more to do with your circadian clock than with differing hyperarousal levels. If you were perfectly adapted to night shift work, you would actually have more problems getting to sleep immediately afterward, too. But this is rarely the case for a variety of reasons, including your quite understandable habit of joining the rest of the world on your days off, as well as the fact that the sun is rising when you leave work.

Some types of night shift workers—emergency room nurses, for example—generate intense hyperarousal. Fighting sleepiness on the job is not a problem in the ER! By contrast, work that requires close monitoring of equipment readouts or security screens cannot be counted on to recruit hyperarousal to fend off sleepiness. Of course, most jobs will fall somewhere between these two extremes. Whatever level of hyperarousal *your* job triggers, you can count on bringing it home and into bed with you in the morning, just as we've seen with evening shift workers. However, at the end of a night shift, your circadian clock is yielding core body temperature and hormonal conditions that are much more conducive to sleep than those that occur in the late evening. These circadian factors often successfully counter hyperarousal, at least at the beginning of your sleep period, in a way that evening shift workers cannot depend on.

HYPERAROUSED BY CHOICE

Most of you reading this chapter do not work either the second or graveyard shift. Neither is it likely that you suffer from idiopathic insomnia, which, fortunately, is not very common. Your hyperarousal is primarily the result of voluntary choices, whether made knowingly, as when you engage in stimulating activities too close to bedtime, or due to misconceptions about how the mechanisms regulating your sleep function.

With regard to your choice of warfare games and horror films prior to bed, you're likely convinced they have no bearing on your sleep. You've probably gone without them a few nights and still had sleep problems. Yes, we acknowledge there is likely more to do to address your insomnia than merely abstaining from such entertainments. Even so, if you're having trouble sleeping, these choices are *still* getting in your way. Tapering off your level of late-night stimulation, as detailed in the next section, will render other interventions more effective.

In terms of misconceptions, one we hear often is that engaging full-throttle in some stimulating late-night activity "wears me out" before bedtime, which in turn leads to sleep. This is generally not a good practice, even if some people possess the genes to get away with it. It usually creates the same conditions of hyperarousal we see in shift workers, without the recompense of a paycheck!

This advice also applies when you fall asleep quickly but find yourself wide awake just a few hours later. You might think that your ability to fall asleep clears your evening activities of any wrongdoing. Not so. You may be able to sleep for a couple of hours even when you have not wound down properly, if you've built up a big enough "sleep debt" across the waking day. The problem is that part of your brain is still "revved up" under that sleep, like an engine gunning in neutral. Once a portion of this sleep debt is paid back and the homeostatic pressure to sleep subsides, residual hyperarousal can still wreak havoc on the rest of your night.

You might be wondering how hyperarousal can persist across several hours of sleep. Isn't sleep the ultimate relaxing activity, automatically setting arousal (and hyperarousal) levels back to zero? Actually, it does not. Remember that the homeostatic sleep drive, the circadian alerting force, and the on-call hyperarousal response are independent, competing mechanisms. Just because one is at a high level (and behaviorally manifest at a given time) does not mean that the others *must* be at low levels. They may just be biding their time. This leads to an important consideration: the best time to relax, to dissipate hyperarousal, *is when you are still awake!* If you fall asleep as if off a cliff, only to awaken a few hours later, it likely means you are not giving yourself adequate time to wind down before bed.

Another common misconception is that one should strictly limit activity throughout the *entire* evening, so as to be absolutely calm before bedtime. Poor sleepers know just how hard it is to stop on a dime at lights out, but this takes things too far. We have treated patients who essentially have no life after work. They will not go out to dinner with friends, or enjoy an evening's walk, expressly because they fear the consequences for sleep. Some will watch TV in a recliner all evening, others will read on the couch, and a few will actually climb into bed at 7 P.M., even though any sleep is likely five or six hours away! Regardless of strategy, the outcome is predictable: they indeed relax during their long hours of stillness, and might even occasionally dip into microsleeps, but when nighttime finally arrives they often get a "second wind" and are not sleepy in the least!

RIDING THE WAVE OF ALERTNESS

At this point you may be thinking, "Okay, I can't be too active, but I also can't get too comfortable. So what *should* I be doing in the evening?" The broad answer to this very reasonable question is that ideally you should match your activity level to your endogenous circadian clock. We'll get into specifics about what that means in a moment, but first just a quick detour into the science underlying our recommendations:

More than thirty-five years ago Charles Czeisler and colleagues discovered that when subjects were experimentally isolated from the twenty-four-hour light/dark cycle caused by the Earth's rotation, when they had no windows to look out of, or mechanical clocks to refer to, a relationship between *when* they slept, according to their circadian clocks, and *how much* they slept could be discerned. Going to bed when those clocks were yielding low core body temperatures led to short sleeps. Going to bed as core temperatures peaked led to long sleeps. In the real world, good sleepers split the difference, going to bed a few hours after their temperature peaks.

A key finding of biological rhythms research in the context of our present discussion is that the core body temperature peak, and therefore our peak level of alertness, *does not occur in the middle of the day.* That is, the circadian alerting force is not a simple sine wave, rising to its highest level at the midpoint of our waking hours. Imagine a hypothetical perfect sleeper who awakens like clockwork at 7 A.M. and falls asleep without fail at 11 P.M., yielding exactly sixteen hours of wakefulness. Her peak level of alertness would not occur eight hours after rising, at 3 P.M. (In fact, due to a circadian rhythm perturbation, she might actually feel a bit sleepy then!) Rather, her alerting force would peak somewhere around 8 P.M.—that is, not all that many hours before she would be sound asleep again.

Though you are not even close to a perfect sleeper, this schematic still holds. To get your best sleep, ride the circadian wave of alertness rather than trying to buck it. Gradually adjust your levels of physical and mental activity in the hours before bedtime to peak in the early evening, and then fall off for a few hours. This will impart the most momentum to your entry into sleep.

In practice, this means that if you too are aiming for an 11 P.M. bedtime, you will want to be highly engaged at 5, 6, and 7 P.M. Preparing a meal and cleaning up afterward or enjoying a dinner out with friends would qualify here, but so would more strenuous activities such as going to the gym, working around the yard, or finishing up household chores. By the hours of 8 and 9 P.M. you will want to be moderately engaged in terms of physical exertion, social stimulation, and cognitive challenge. You may be getting children off to bed, helping with homework, doing last rounds of email and social networking, paying bills, or watching a favorite show. You do not want to be doing any heavy lifting, either literally or figuratively. Finally, you should set aside a "buffer period" for the last hour or two before bedtime. This is the time to turn off all your interactive, socially connective electronic devices "in preparation for landing." Try curling up in a chair with a book under a reading lamp, listening to serene music, or just having a quiet conversation.

We know that most of you are in front of television, laptop, or phone screens in the last hours before bed, or even while in your bed. You've tried reading or listening to soothing music many times in the past, and by now are certain that such activities can't hold your attention for more than fifteen minutes. This is to be expected, given that you are prone to hyperarousal. For you, the rapid-fire editing of television and films, the hair-trigger suspense of video games, and the endless links offered by the internet will always prove much more satisfying. You must come to understand, however, that your immersion in fast-paced media in the hours before bedtime is not just a risk factor for insomnia in general. *It is the first phase of tonight's sleeplessness.*

A touchstone of our approach is that the quality of your night's sleep is in large part *already decided* by the time you turn off the light. So, the best time for making decisions and taking actions is beforehand, not afterward. We encourage you to begin making a change tonight, by reading *anything*—book, magazine, newspaper, comic, catalog, or brochure—for ten to fifteen minutes before bedtime. Gradually, you may grow to tolerate reading for twenty or thirty minutes. If you prefer listening, choose quiet music, an audiobook, or a podcast, rather than talk radio or top-forty stations that interject attention-grabbing commercials every three minutes. Our aim here is not to make you a better reader or listener, but a better sleeper. Still, since sleep and wakefulness are two phases of a single cycle, you can't really change one without changing the other.

SOME RELAXATION IS BETTER THAN NONE

So far we've emphasized the selection and timing of *habitual* activities to match your underlying alertness cycle. After all, you won't stay with an activity if you don't like doing it. Some of you may have to expand your behavioral repertoire to fill the final waking phase, the buffer period before sleep. The one new practice we would advise *all* of you to adopt, given your history of hyperarousal, is that of *relaxation training*.

We are well aware that we are venturing here into treacherous terrain. If there is one thing you cannot tolerate, and perhaps even find hateful, it is "trying to relax." Just hearing the phrase may conjure up an image of your body getting antsy and your mind beginning to race, as you try to "do nothing" for what seems an eternity.

Actually, traditional relaxation training, as described in chapter 1, does "do something" specifically tailored to your needs: it teaches you to *recognize your hyperarousal*, whatever its baseline level, and focus on the part that can be soothed. Relaxation training also gives you tools to bring your hyperarousal down. Whether in the form of muscle tension, shallow breathing, mind racing, or other symptoms, its level at any given time (a combination of trait and state components), is not set in stone. You can learn to live with less.

What about your antsiness and distractibility? How can you possibly calm yourself when you are so keyed into barking dogs, drafty rooms, traffic noise, pillows that are too hard or too soft, and other intrusions? Try practicing the following technique, which we have employed for many years to help people like you. It's best applied after you have prepared the way with traditional treatments such as progressive relaxation or deep breathing exercises, even if you can attain only a halfway relaxed state through such means.

Imagine you are watching a parade. You have secured a particularly good vantage point. There is no reason to move at all; you can see and hear the entire spectacle from just where you are. This parade is not made up of floats and marching bands—it is an "everyday" parade but it still presents an unending progression of things passing by. After a while you grow tired, and close your eyes.

You can still hear and feel everything: Two people converse as they walk outside. A fly buzzes near the window. The refrigerator starts up its cycle. A police siren passes about two blocks away. A wave of warmth emanates from the radiator. The house creaks.

The parade route extends through your mind: A reminder that you should pick up a carton of milk for the morning wafts by. You wonder about the final tally for your car in the shop. There's a dream snippet from last night, clear as a movie trailer! What was that mistake you made on the spreadsheet yesterday?

True, on occasion one of your parade's participants may turn out to be something important to remember. If you wish, once you have finished your review you can jot down a note about it for the next day. But you'll soon grow to appreciate that most of the thoughts are trivial, most of the irritants transient. Your task, such as it is, is merely to watch them come and go. The point of this exercise is not to become more observant of the world outside, nor to become more adept at dredging up the contents of your mind. It is simply to cultivate detachment, to find the gear labeled *neutral,* to learn that sometimes there is nothing you need respond to at all.

EXERCISE AND HYPERAROUSAL

Apart from its many other benefits, exercise has been shown to reduce hyperarousal and to improve insomnia. While your nonrestorative sleep and wired wakefulness do not likely provide much of an inducement for you to work out, we nonetheless recommend regular, moderate physical exertion (unless contraindicated by your physician). As with many of the other recommendations in this book, we understand that we are asking you to sustain an effort before its benefits for sleep become apparent. Such is often the case when attempting to break a vicious cycle. Over time you may find that healthy routines become self-sustaining, as you enjoy increased fitness and well-being, not to mention calmer waking hours and improved sleep.

Your choice of exercise should take into account both its physical demands and your level of motivation. While there has been relatively limited systematic work in the area of exercise and sleep, several studies showing positive results employed moderate aerobic exercise—for example, thirty or forty-five minutes on a treadmill. The best time of day for exercise in terms of effect on sleep also appears to vary between individuals. The bulk of the scientific literature points to deeper sleep resulting from exercising in the late afternoon or early evening, at least four hours before bedtime. A minority of individuals report that later evening exercise is helpful, whereas most people are too revved up by such activity. Finally, if early morning happens to be the time you can most reliably set aside for a workout, go for it. Long-term studies have shown benefits on sleep from early morning exercise (perhaps mediated by a general improvement in fitness). In any case, damping down hyperarousal right from the start of your day may well prove beneficial in its own right.

HYPERAROUSAL AND PTSD

To conclude this chapter, we offer words of encouragement and advice specifically to those of you who are contending with hyperarousal reactive to trauma. First off, we should emphasize that many of the recommendations we made to shift workers and to those whose voluntary evening choices predispose them to insomnia can help you as well. You, too, should make sure there is an adequate interval between strenuous or overstimulating activities and bedtime. You, too, should strive to match your level of engagement in the evening to the lateness of the hour, starting from an early evening peak and gradually becoming more sedentary and buffered from the day's demands.

However, you differ in what it takes for you to feel sufficiently secure at night. For example, you may feel more at ease after conducting a perimeter check, or when sleeping in a front room of the house that allows for a view of the street. Traditional relaxation exercises may well make you jumpy or trigger flashbacks rather than calming you down. Don't hesitate to pick and choose any interventions that keep your hyperarousal at bay. We are not striving here for total peace and tranquility. Ratcheting down your stress level just a few notches will help.

But frankly, all this may not be enough. If you suspect you have PTSD, we advise that you seek professional evaluation. There are now targeted, evidence-based treatments, both behavioral and pharmacological, for your condition that can directly address your symptoms. In terms of improving sleep, your treatment plan will likely require formal CBT-I, provided by a specialist, and possibly medication as well. The specifics of your treatment regimen will, of course, be decided within the collaboration you undertake with your providers. Here we offer some general observations, gained through years of clinical experience, which may prove useful in your discussions.

In chapter 1 we reviewed sleep restriction therapy

(SRT), a treatment for insomnia originated in 1987 that has since established itself as a core component of CBT-I. Over the years we have written numerous articles and chapters describing its presumed mechanisms, applications, and effects. One of these effects has direct application to you: although many patients have difficulty contending with the daytime sleepiness that is a common initial side effect of SRT, the treatment is often *better* tolerated by those with hyperarousal.

We don't have to tell you that daytime sleepiness is generally not one of your problems, even though you hardly ever sleep well at night. Hyperarousal is very effective when it comes to opposing sleepiness—but the opposite holds as well. Sleepiness generated by SRT seems to mitigate hyperarousal. Of course, there is a limit to how much extra sleep drive can be introduced, but if titrated properly, SRT can take the edge off the way you feel by day, while at night it works to deepen and consolidate sleep.

We emphasized above that the quality of your night's sleep is determined by the nature of the preceding hours of wakefulness. This has an important ramification for those of you who are considering pharmacological treatment. If left unchecked, the heightened arousal you bring into bed can overwhelm hypnotic medication taken just fifteen or thirty minutes beforehand. Some of our patients seem to have intuited this, and they may resort to taking sleeping pills several hours before their intended bedtime "to give them a chance to work."

This is not how hypnotic medications are intended to be used. This practice can lead to unpleasant feelings of dissociation or "being out of it," as well as overt sleepiness and an increased risk of falls. In addition, today's hypnotics are formulated to be relatively short acting, so you may end up going to bed just as the sleep-inducing effect of the pill you took has peaked. Your provider may consider other classes of medication, including certain antianxiety drugs and antidepressants, which can safely and effectively address hyperarousal during the critical hours before bedtime, in this way helping prepare you for sleep.

From our point of view this approach has the added benefit of weakening the association between taking a pill and going to sleep. While we will be covering the topic of medication thoroughly in a later chapter, here we will just say that people who take hypnotic medication tend to give most of the credit for any sleep they achieve to the pills. By contrast, using medication to promote relaxed wakefulness in the hours before bedtime still requires the final approach into sleep to be "flown solo" and makes explicit the collaborative nature between you and your medication in reaching your goal of restful sleep.

Though we have encouraged those of you who struggle with posttraumatic hyperarousal to seek professional help, we do not want to imply that your prognosis is poor. We have seen the sleep of veterans, disturbed since the war in Vietnam, respond to CBT-I treatment within a few months. We have seen incest survivors, hypervigilant since childhood, find a measure of repose at night. If you can remember a time when you slept adequately, even if it was decades ago, we are confident that better sleep can be in your future, too.

CHAPTER SUMMARY

- Hyperarousal is an "emergency override" system, sometimes erupting within seconds. It keeps us alert when falling asleep would be dangerous. From an evolutionary standpoint this makes good sense. However, hyperarousal can also be triggered by situations that are not true emergencies, such as when working conditions prove too demanding, or just when worry about sleeplessness gets out of hand. It can then take hours to subside.

- Some of you are prone to hyperarousal by nature, while others have acquired a tendency to hyperarousal through traumatic experience. In either case, it now takes less of a disturbance or threat to elicit this response. Once hyperarousal is triggered, it takes you longer to return to your baseline arousal level, and longer to drift off from there to sleep.

- Whether hyperarousal results from work stress or just a stimulating evening, the most effective way to address it is by inserting a "buffer period" of relaxed wakefulness, of at least one hour, before bedtime. This is especially important if you are coming off an evening shift (because the circadian clock is still strongly promoting wakefulness during these hours). For you, a buffer period is a good tradeoff, even though it means your bedtime will be extra late.

- Just because you manage to fall asleep does not mean that your hyperarousal has been adequately addressed. The buildup of homeostatic sleep drive over a long day may allow you to doze off, even as hyperarousal continues to churn underneath. This often leads to just an hour or two of sleep (paying off the worst of the sleep debt) and then rousing with a start. You cannot really relax in sleep; that's something you must find time to do while still awake.

- Some of you do not find peace and quiet particularly pleasant. You may get antsy or anxious when trying to relax with books or music, preferring faster-paced diversions. Tearing apart an engine or playing games on the phone may be fine for earlier in the evening. However, you would do well to learn to tolerate progressively longer stints of reading or listening right before bedtime. Think of your discomfort with relaxation as the opening act of tonight's insomnia. It should also be treated with behavioral interventions.

- If your hyperarousal stems from posttraumatic stress disorder, you may benefit from specialized psychotherapeutic strategies and medication, in addition to following the guidelines presented in this chapter. Assuring that both your inner and outer worlds are sufficiently safeguarded is crucial, for ultimately you are the only one who can decide that it is okay to sleep.

CHAPTER THREE

Are You **Fatigued** Instead of Sleepy?

FATIGUE AND SLEEPINESS ARE NOT THE SAME THING

How can one be fatigued yet not sleepy? At first glance it doesn't make much sense. Indeed, many people use the words interchangeably, and the English language doesn't help matters when the word "tired" can be used as a synonym for each. However, whether one probes further into dictionary definitions or human physiology, there are clear differences to be found. In short, *fatigue* implies weariness from some physical or mental effort, whereas *sleepiness* means drowsiness—the propensity to fall and stay asleep. People who are fatigued tend to rest, while those who are sleepy tend to sleep.

This may sound like splitting hairs to some, but not to those of you who know from firsthand experience just how demoralizing it is to suffer debilitating fatigue by day, and then be restless, rather than sleepy, at night. You've paid your dues, in the sense of having plodded through endless hours with your motivation sapped, your limbs exhausted, and your mind befuddled. Wakefulness has been one long, gargantuan effort. Why won't it draw to a close?

The reason you're not getting your nightly allotment of sleep, if you're counting on fatigue to bring it to you, is that you've been waiting in the wrong line! Your confusion is understandable, since for many of us the goal of "feeling good" during waking hours means being neither sleepy nor fatigued. Moreover, you may remember better times when, after putting in a full day's work, you were both sleepy and fatigued. This is probably what led you to blur the two states in the first place. You thought that if you got one, you got the other.

Of course, once we have defined our terms, it becomes clear that you are living proof that one can indeed be fatigued without being sleepy. The opposite also holds true: There are many people who are quite sleepy without complaining of being particularly fatigued. Not having exerted themselves, either physically or mentally, they are often surprised and frustrated when, in the midst of watching a favorite show, they fall asleep.

Your fatigue may be of unclear origin, or tied to conditions as diverse as nutritional deficiency, cancer, hormone imbalance, fibromyalgia, infection, or autoimmune disorder. Whatever the case, we trust that you and your healthcare providers are working closely to monitor and address this often debilitating symptom. What we can bring to the mix is a vantage point that is often overlooked—one that emphasizes the interaction of fatigue with both sleep and wakefulness.

This view brings considerable practical benefit. For while sleepiness and fatigue are not interchangeable, they may still *influence* each other: contending with chronic fatigue by day can affect your propensity for sleep at night, while the quality of your sleep may in turn modify your fatigue, for better or worse. We will be proposing specific cognitive and behavioral interventions to take advantage of this leverage, to both increase your sleepiness at night and decrease your daytime fatigue.

SLEEPINESS AT NIGHT REFLECTS YOUR WAKING HOURS

To feel sleepy at night, your homeostatic sleep drive must be elevated. This is why waking hours are so important to sleep. Your sleep drive increases with each passing hour of wakefulness, just as hunger increases as time goes by without food. It doesn't much matter when that wakefulness accumulates—it can be the intentional wakefulness you count on during the day to get your work done. Or it can be the unwelcome wakefulness of insomnia. Waking hours—at any time—boost your sleep drive.

What does matter, however, is that in those hours you are *fully* awake. If your fatigue leads you to spend many hours in a recliner or bed, your sleep drive will not increase as much as if you had spent those hours more actively engaged. This is the case even when, from your perspective, you remained awake the whole time. For, just as some sleep is "better," in terms of depth and consolidation, wakefulness varies in quality as well. Extended wakefulness in a recliner, let alone a bed, turns out to be not very awake at all.

When you slow down to rest, your brain waves also slow down. The fast, low-voltage beta activity of alertness and cognitive engagement, with frequencies of about 14 to 35 cycles per second (also known as "Hertz" or Hz), begins to drop out. If you happen to close your eyes you may begin to produce alpha waves, EEG activity of 8 to 12 Hz, characteristic of relaxed wakefulness. Even if your eyes remain open, after a while you may start to have *microsleeps*—periods of actual EEG sleep, now including activity down to the theta range of about 4 to 7 Hz, persisting for a few seconds.

This EEG slowing and brief dipping into sleep reduces your sleep drive, even though subjectively you may feel certain you "didn't really sleep." If your bedrest becomes extended, with too much time spent lingering about the border between wakefulness and sleep, you may be on your way to experiencing the worst of both worlds—unable to enjoy a brief, refreshing nap by day, and then unable to sleep soundly later on.

So the unfortunate truth is that the very thing that eases your fatigue by day—resting comfortably—detracts from your ability to sleep well at night. We know what a quandary this raises, and will have suggestions on how to strike the right balance, for your particular circumstances, in the second half of this chapter. Here, we just set out the problem as one that somehow needs to be addressed if you are to be ready for sleep at night.

DAYTIME FATIGUE MAY REFLECT HOW WELL YOU SLEPT

We don't have to tell you that when it comes to chronic fatigue, you have better days and worse days, sometimes for no clear-cut reason. For example, if your exhaustion is associated with multiple sclerosis, you no doubt understand that fatigue is a very common symptom of the disorder, but may still wonder how it can vary so widely from one day to the next, even when your other MS symptoms are stable. Fatigue is a complex physiological state, reflecting numerous factors. The quality of your sleep is only one of these. However, because the quality of sleep varies greatly, literally from night to night, it can play an outsized role in determining how you feel on a given day. It also presents a particularly ripe target for intervention.

For most of you, the problem is not one of getting enough sleep. Your bedtime schedule is not squeezed between work and morning obligations, like the evening shift workers we considered in our chapter on hyperarousal. Generally, you can set aside enough hours—you just cannot fill them with quality sleep. Either it is full of holes, in the sense of its being interrupted by full-blown awakenings, or you awaken in the morning with the perception that you were "half asleep" the entire night.

When the problem is one of full-blown awakenings, the culprit is usually once again a diminished homeostatic sleep drive. Waking up for a few seconds now and then during sleep—known as a *transient arousal*—is normal. It generally happens a few dozen times in a night without our awareness, and without significant daytime consequences. However, if your sleep drive is reduced, it becomes harder to be pulled back into sleep, once you have roused. As the seconds stretch out to minutes, your mind will of course start to come up with of all kinds of thoughts demanding attention, and then you may be awake for hours.

Chronic fatigue is more commonly associated with sleep that, while covering most of the night, is nonetheless perceived as light and nonrestorative. Here, the problem is one of *quality* rather than quantity. What does this poor-quality sleep look like?

Poor sleep may be riddled with an excessive number of the same transient arousals just mentioned above. Instead of just a few dozen, a single night of sleep may contain a hundred or more transient arousals. These arousals are often associated with specific sleep disturbances such as obstructive sleep apnea or periodic leg movements in sleep. They can also result from a host of other causes, such as chronic pain, environmental noise, or poorly regulated body temperature. Finally, they may appear for no clear reason at all, in which case they are termed *spontaneous arousals*. Most investigations into the matter have explored the relationship between transient arousals and overt daytime sleepiness. However, a smaller body of literature has also linked these arousals to increased fatigue.

Another transient change in the EEG, one that is specifically associated with daytime fatigue, is known as an *alpha intrusion*. These are bursts of the same 8 to 12 Hz alpha activity discussed above in the context of relaxed wakefulness, but now riding on top of the slower waves of NREM sleep. While the link between alpha activity and wakefulness may suggest that alpha intrusions in sleep represent a sort of incomplete awakening, they are not associated with brief movements in bed or even an increase in muscle tone, as is often seen with transient arousals. Behaviorally, the sleeper stays asleep, and other aspects of the polysomnographic record remain unchanged. The sole perceived consequence may be exacerbated daytime fatigue.

Poor sleep associated with fatigue can also be characterized by changes in *sleep architecture*. For example, sleep may contain an excessive amount of light transitional NREM stage 1 sleep, a stage from which, if people are awakened, they may well report that they were not sleeping at all! It may be characterized by an absence or reduction of the deepest, most restorative NREM stage, stage 3. This stage contains large, rolling *delta waves*, typically less than 2 Hz, which arise from synchronization in the firing rate of large numbers of neurons—indicating a brain truly at rest.

Finally, sleep architecture may be altered by an excessive number of sleep *stage changes*. We usually have four or five NREM/REM cycles per night, and as we make our way through these cycles we can easily rack up forty or fifty shifts between the stages of wakefulness, NREM sleep stages 1, 2 and 3, and REM sleep. When sleep architecture is particularly disturbed, it is not uncommon to see three or four times as many stage changes as usual. If these stage shifts are toward wakefulness and NREM stage 1 sleep, daytime fatigue is a predictable result.

In each of these cases—whether sleep is marred by excessive transient arousals, alpha intrusions, or disturbances of sleep architecture—it is perceived as shallow and unrefreshing. You wake up feeling like you've "been run over by a truck." You have likely used a 0-to-10 rating scale to rate your fatigue in working with your doctors. When fatigue has been hovering around 5 or 6 and then, without any other perceived flare-up in illness, registers an 8 or 9, diminished sleep quality is often at least partly to blame.

FATIGUE WILL NOT GET YOU TO SLEEP

We have emphasized that fatigue and sleepiness are quite distinct. In some ways, fatigue may be thought of as the more complex state, as it involves basic metabolic and immune processes that affect much of our physiology at the cellular level. Fatigue is also associated with a wide array of medical conditions. By contrast, normal sleepiness may be viewed as a relatively narrow, mechanistic response to sleep loss. Its main purpose may be to get us to seek out our next sleep opportunity as soon as we can, and sleep more soundly when it comes! Indeed, this is the essence of the homeostatic mechanism of sleep regulation. As the "enforcement arm" of this mechanism, sleepiness works in concert with the circadian clock to get us in a good position for sleep, both literally and figuratively, when the right time rolls around.

Fatigue is not integral to sleep regulation in this way. As noted at the outset of this discussion, it leads to rest, not to sleep. And rest is not tightly governed by the circadian clock. *Unlike sleep, rest can be obtained more or less at will, at any time of day or night.*

This is no doubt counted as good news by you who are burdened with chronic fatigue. Imagine how much more difficult your life would be if rest were as elusive as sleep, if you could not count on being able to rest when you needed to. (Actually, some readers, such as those contending with chronic pain, may be in just such a predicament.) While there is a definite advantage to your being able to rest as needed, this handy remedy comes at a cost: excessive bedrest diminishes your sleep drive without bringing the benefits of sleep. Furthermore, when that bedrest is scattered across all hours of the day, it blunts the circadian sleep/wake cycle. The upshot is that not only does your fatigue not lead to sleep, your quest to cope with that fatigue may well be perpetuating insomnia.

· · ·

Where does all of this leave you, who contend with chronic and severe fatigue? We know that it is not your choice to reduce your activity level, to interrupt your life with rest periods. You likely settled upon this coping strategy through trial and error, after learning how much of a price you paid when you pushed yourself too hard. You may be convinced that the present level of functioning is the best you can do, under the circumstances.

We of course have no knowledge of the origins of your fatigue, its intensity, or how well you are dealing with it. We cannot take into account your age, daily obligations, physical condition, medical status, or other factors known to affect fatigue. However, now that we have traced a link between resting to compensate for fatigue and difficulty sleeping, we can offer specific suggestions to manage your fatigue in ways that are more compatible with sleeping well.

Each of you will have to work out how these suggestions might apply to your particular circumstances. Before you make any changes we recommend that you consult with your physician to discuss whether *any* increase in your level of activity or structuring of your rest periods is advisable. Certainly some medical conditions dictate either prolonged bedrest or rest whenever you feel the need. You may also wish to discuss your plans with other members of the household, whose own routines may be affected by the changes you introduce, and whose support can prove invaluable when you are trying to break long-established patterns.

LEARNING **HOW** TO REST

For those who get the go-ahead, we ask in essence that you stop resting by default—that you stop thinking of rest as something that just happens when you are too fatigued to do anything else—and instead start making decisions about *how to rest*. As silly as it might sound when discussing something that has come naturally your whole life, you will want to learn how to rest in a more considered, intentional way. In this, the situation is the exact opposite of what we have proposed for sleep, which at the end of the day should be a no-brainer. The key difference is that you can't summon sleep at will, but you can in fact summon rest. Therefore you need to be more prudent about when you do.

We may be in danger of losing some of you right here, those who are convinced that your fatigue leaves you no choice but to lie down and rest. Indeed, fatigue can at times be overwhelming. We just ask that you decide when, and to what extent, you are able to follow these guidelines:

1. Rest at the **Right Time**

Many of you tend to rest in bed during the morning. This is usually because you've had a restless night and are feeling rotten. You need to collect yourself, to marshal your limited energy for the long day ahead. On the other hand, you may rest in the morning simply because it feels good to stay in your warm, comfortable bed. While everyone else has to deal with the weather, the traffic, and the hubbub outside their bedroom windows as day begins, you have no pressing engagement.

Others will climb into bed early in the evening, well before you have much chance of falling into a deep sleep that could conceivably carry through the night. Again, there are two main reasons why you do: Most of the time you feel completely drained by the day just passed—and you'll take whatever you can get in terms of sleep, dozing, restfulness, or just getting off your feet! At other times getting into bed early is more of a choice—one of life's few pleasures. It's a time to read or watch TV, to play with that new app on your phone, or listen to music. Evening bedrest can feel like a brief vacation, a well-earned reward for making it through another day. However, whether it represents a choice or not, prolonged rest in the morning *or* in the evening, adjacent to when you actually try to sleep at night, dims your prospects for sleeping well.

This is so because getting into bed for protracted stretches before you turn out the light, or staying cocooned long after you have awakened, will weaken your sleep drive, disrupt the timing of your circadian clock, and loosen the association you have learned to make between being in bed and sleeping. Even if your intention is to "just rest," excessive time in bed potentially engages and disrupts these mechanisms regulating your ability to sleep.

In the evening, a direct hit is taken by your homeostatic sleep drive. The mere act of lying down has important physiological consequences: Your postural muscles relax. Your blood pressure and heart rate decrease. There are changes in the distribution of heat between your trunk and your extremities so that your fingers and toes begin to warm and midbrain sleep centers are activated. When you close your eyes and start dipping into microsleeps you really start to spread your sleep drive thin. The result is broken sleep with longer sleep latencies, more interspersed wakefulness once you do fall asleep, and more time spent in lighter rather than deeper stages of NREM sleep.

Resting in bed during the morning hours not only

squanders sleep drive, it also dampens your circadian rhythms. Your sleep/wake rhythm is strongest when you sleep deeply in a dark, quiet, cool environment for a fairly regular duration, ending at the same time each twenty-four-hour cycle, and then get out of bed—preferably to go outdoors. This allows for a predictable, abrupt transition between darkness and light, which is *the most effective way to set the circadian clock.* A habit of resting in the morning for an hour or two, whether with eyes closed or just squirreled away from daylight, is therefore particularly disruptive.

So when should you allow yourself a rest period if you decide you need one? For a typical nighttime sleep pattern, the best time to do so is generally in the early to midafternoon, somewhere near the middle of your waking hours. If you rise at 7:30 A.M. and go to bed at 10:30 P.M., for example, your waking day is fifteen hours long. A good time to rest would be about seven-and-a-half hours after rising, or around 3 P.M. An hour-long rest period would therefore be between 2:30 and 3:30 P.M.

This timing has the advantage of breaking up the day into manageable segments. It also accords well with our circadian clock, which tends to produce a dip in alertness twelve hours out of phase with the middle of the main sleep period. In the above example, the sleep period extends over nine hours from 10:30 P.M. to 7:30 A.M., with a midpoint of 3 A.M., hence the afternoon dip around 3 P.M. Siesta cultures have long taken advantage of the biologically based nook for afternoon sleep in conjunction with a relatively short nocturnal sleep phase, albeit usually on a later all-around schedule than the one discussed here.

WHEN YOU NEED MORE REST

Some of you cannot make it through the day with just one period for rest. If you feel the need for two, it is still important that you avoid bedrest at either end of your waking day. In practice, this will mean that you have one rest period in the late morning and another a bit later in the afternoon than the time suggested above, perhaps centering on 4:30 P.M. instead of 3 P.M. This will break your day into three active segments, and still keep you out of bed or off the couch for at least five or six hours before turning in for the night.

Finally, we would like to direct a few words to those of you who are sedentary nearly the entire day. Such extended inactivity can be the clear consequence of many medical illnesses and physical disabilities; it may also be reactive to fatigue that has a poorly understood cause. In either case, it is likely that you are not catching much quality sleep, despite casting such a wide net in terms of time in bed. We assume you are working with your doctors to optimize your mobility and activity level. In a minority of cases enforced bedrest is medically advised, and of course this recommendation takes precedence over our suggestions. For the rest of you, imposing some structure, as best you can, on the timing of your sleep, rest, and activity will pay off both in terms of better nighttime sleep and daytime functioning.

In *The Insomnia Answer* we introduced the concept of "sleep-free zones" to readers whose sleep was spread haphazardly, in short stints, across the twenty-four hours of the day. These sleep-free zones were designated hours, however few, in which readers agreed to stay out of bed. They were also asked to avoid dozing wherever else they might find themselves when inside the zone. For example, sleep-free zones might consist of three hours in the morning from 8 A.M. to 11 A.M., and three hours in the evening from 8 P.M. to 11 P.M., when sleep would not happen. During the remaining eighteen hours of each cycle, readers who required this intervention *would be free to sleep or not*. Gradually the duration of the sleep-free zones would be increased, to the point where most daytime hours would be spent awake, perhaps leaving time for one or two naps.

The same concept can be helpful for you who rest much of the day, whether on a bed, couch, or recliner. Designate two or three hours, right before bedtime and also upon arising, as "rest-free zones." During the morning zone you should aim to be relatively active and get your various chores done. During the evening zone you can include more passive options such as watching TV, reading, or listening to music, seated in a comfortable chair. During the remainder of the day you are free to rest, with the provision that this does not mean you should automatically climb into bed. The *ways* in which you rest should vary depending upon your fatigue level, as we will soon discuss. Gradually, you may increase the duration of your rest-free zones, and carve out a third zone in the middle of the day

Some of you may be wondering what's so different about this plan, compared to your usual behavior. You often mobilize as best you can for a few hours, when you are feeling up to it, to get things done or find some enjoyment. The difference is that by responding to an external clock rather than the vagaries of how you feel at a given moment, you will be indirectly strengthening your circadian sleep/wake cycle. In timing rest periods more rigorously, you thereby regulate *activity* as well. The "wake" portion of your sleep/wake cycle will be strengthened, becoming more differentiated from the sleep phase. Your chances of being exposed to bright light during the morning hours will be increased. All of this will in turn lead to deeper, more refreshing sleep at night.

2. Rest for the **Right Amount of Time**

In the example above we cite a rest period of one hour. There is nothing especially beneficial about this duration. Some people do well with short breaks of ten or twenty minutes, while others require more extended bedrest. Moreover, an individual's need for rest will vary across time. What we suggest is that you are mindful of the intensity of your fatigue, and rest just enough to resume modest activity. Note that you are likely to err on the side of resting too much, simply because unlike sleep, how long you rest is completely up to you. So, if you typically stay in bed for about an hour and a half, set a timer to prompt consideration of rising after an hour, or even forty-five minutes. The goal is to take the edge off your fatigue, not to be as "well rested" as possible.

3. Match the **Depth of Your Rest** to the Intensity of your Fatigue

The distinction between "light sleep" and "deep sleep" is probably both familiar and intuitive. That sleep varies in depth has also found experimental confirmation. As sleepers progress through NREM stages 1, 2, and 3, they become more difficult to rouse. (REM sleep is a special case in this regard. It is sometimes called "paradoxical sleep" because its EEG resembles that of the waking state. It can nonetheless be difficult at times to rouse someone from REM sleep, in part because interruptions tend to be incorporated into the ongoing dream activity characteristic of this stage.)

We don't often differentiate between "light rest" and "deep rest," but in the context of this discussion perhaps we should. Lying in bed is not the *only* way to rest. In fact, it qualifies as one of its deepest forms, and should be reserved for special occasions, given how detrimental it can be to your sleep drive and circadian rhythms. Some mild forms of activity may also qualify as "rest," in the sense that they would not at that moment present much of a mental or physical challenge. For example, if your fatigue level is at 6 out of 10, you still may be able to play cards or thumb through a magazine. This qualifies as resting even though you are not in bed.

Or say you have really exerted yourself, perhaps with some yard work or by cleaning up the kitchen. Sipping a beverage in an easy chair may allow you to regroup sufficiently to stay out of bed. You might then turn to some modest activity such as folding clothes or paying bills, whereas if you had just plopped yourself down out of exhaustion you might soon be whiling away hours in a twilight state.

We do not mean to imply that your goal is to *always* be active. Sometimes it will make sense for you to just climb into bed—you'll know when that is the case. The key point is that it should be a *considered decision*, which takes into account the severity of your fatigue, the likely effect of bed-rest at that hour on your subsequent prospects for sleep, the viability of other restful options and, if the decision is to lie down, the amount of time needed to enable resumption of modest activity. If you are mindful and judicious in allotting yourself bedrest, you can learn to optimize rest, just as you strive to optimize sleep. Both your nights and days will be more refreshing as a result.

CHAPTER SUMMARY

- Although *fatigued* and *sleepy* are sometimes used interchangeably as synonyms for *tired*, they are not one and the same. *Fatigued* refers to being weary from physical or mental effort. *Sleepy* refers to being drowsy or ready to fall asleep. It's quite possible to be fatigued without being sleepy, as well as to be sleepy without being fatigued.
- The origins of fatigue are complex. When it arises from healthy physical exertion or mental effort it is fully reversible by resting. However, fatigue may also be chronic and associated with a wide array of disorders, including nutritional deficiency, hormone imbalance, infection, fibromyalgia, multiple sclerosis, cancer, and heart disease. To further complicate matters, fatigue is a potential side effect of many medical treatments.
- Sleepiness is generally more straightforward. It is reg-

ulated by a homeostatic sleep drive, which increases sleepiness with each waking hour, and a circadian clock, which counters sleepiness with an alerting force that rises and falls every twenty-four hours. Excessive sleepiness rarely represents a neurological problem. Usually, sleep of inadequate quantity or quality is to blame.

- While fatigue and sleepiness represent independent phenomena, they do interact. When fatigue prompts prolonged periods of bedrest during the day, it can sap the homeostatic sleep drive and blunt the circadian sleep/wake cycle. Inadequate sleep, on the other hand, may inhibit restorative processes at the cellular level, and result in flare-ups of fatigue.

- In contrast to highly regulated sleep, rest can generally be taken at any time, for as long as it is desired. This ready availability, coupled with the detrimental effects excessive bedrest can have on sleep, make it important that you do not rest indiscriminately, unless your doctor recommends otherwise. Funny as it may sound, you would do well to learn how to rest.

- It is important to rest at the right time. In general, this means in the middle of your waking day, when resting will have less chance of throwing off your circadian clock, and when there is still an opportunity to rebuild your homeostatic sleep drive.

- It is also important to rest for the right amount of time. This amount will vary between individuals. However, because the choice is yours to make, you are likely resting more than necessary. You cannot be "as well rested as possible" by day and still sleep well at night.

- Match the depth of your rest to the intensity of your fatigue. Rest, like sleep, can be light or deep. Aim to rest in a way that provides relief but still maintains modest activity and engagement. Save bedrest, the deepest form of rest, for the times when you really need it.

CHAPTER FOUR

Are You Too **Depressed** to Sleep?

"That would be just my rotten luck," you may be thinking, "because all I seem to want to do these days is sleep."

The depression that has enveloped you is densely woven. Weighed down by sadness, isolation, apathy, and futility, to name just a few of its strands, merely getting through the day requires extraordinary effort. It's no wonder you long for sleep. Not that sleeping solves all your problems, but at least it provides a temporary escape. The only glitch is that lately, even something as basic as sleep seems to require more effort than it should. Either you feel too agitated and unsettled to ever reach deep slumber or else you awaken way too early, to face a string of cold, dark hours alone. What should be a haven has instead become just another affliction.

DEPRESSION AND SLEEP
ARE INTERDEPENDENT

Into this bleak scenario we can shine a ray of hope, as something extraordinary has been learned about the relationship between sleep and depression in recent years, thanks to pioneering work by Rachel Manber and her colleagues. Simply put, it's that sleeplessness is not merely a symptom of depression, as we and generations of other clinicians were trained to believe. That is, poor sleep is not something that you simply must endure, that you cannot hope to shake until your depression lifts. Rather, sleep and depression are *interdependent*. Each influences the course of the other. What this means for you is that your hopes for better sleep, starting tonight, are not doomed to failure just because you have a mood disorder. You can *still* position yourself to fall asleep more readily, to sleep more soundly. In turn, better sleep can *alter the course of your depression*.

It has long been known that insomnia and depression commonly appear together, but now we have a better understanding of why this is so. It turns out that sleep and mood are linked in many ways, through both psychological and neurophysiological mechanisms. This interdependence has been hinted at many times over: early morning awakenings are a classic feature of major depression. Another is its *diurnal mood variation*, which refers to a predictable worsening of mood in the morning hours that lifts later in the day. This is essentially a circadian mood disturbance—a blend of depression with the sleep/wake cycle if ever there was one! Finally, research dating back forty-five years demonstrates that sleep deprivation, and in particular REM sleep deprivation, yields clear-cut if temporary antidepressant effects.

Depression interacts with sleep by influencing behavior as well as mood. Some types of depression are described as "agitated," marked by a general restlessness that inhibits sleep directly. In other instances depression is characterized by lethargy and daytime sleepiness, leading to extended periods of sleep, or at least bedrest. Perhaps the clearest demonstration of the linkage between sleep, waking behavior, and depression is provided by bipolar disorder, known informally as "manic-depression," where these factors all track together: protracted wakefulness, hyperactivity, and impulsivity are hallmarks of the manic phase of this disturbance, whereas when the depressive phase sets in, waking hours become lethargic, and the urge to sleep returns—although that urge may be met with either prolonged sleep episodes or the disrupted sleep of insomnia. Yet another direct link between sleep and bipolar disorder is evidenced by the observation that sleep restriction can trigger manic episodes in predisposed individuals.

Besides being apparent to the trained eye, the interrelatedness of sleep and depression is written in our brain waves. As polysomnography became more widely deployed in research and clinical settings more than forty years ago, one of the first things looked at was sleep in various psychiatric conditions. Soon thereafter, the first papers describing predictable alterations of sleep in depression appeared. This work confirmed the presence of generally disrupted sleep and early morning awakenings, as had already been expected on the basis of clinical observation. It also uncovered several intriguing findings regarding REM sleep—the "paradoxical" sleep stage characterized by EEG activation instead of slowing, and by involved dream narratives rather than the blank mind or simple thoughts of NREM sleep. In a word, REM sleep seems more *insistent* in those who are depressed.

For example, REM sleep doesn't wait the usual amount of time after sleep onset before making its first appearance—it jumps the line over NREM stages, leading to the so-called shortened REM latency characteristic of depression. It also contains more of the phasic rapid eye movements that give the sleep stage its name—referred to as a higher "REM density." Moreover, there is a general redistribution of REM sleep from later to earlier hours of sleep. In fact, this "phase advance" of REM has been proposed to account for depression's early morning awakenings. In this view, as REM sleep migrates to earlier hours, it leaves a gap of wakefulness at the end of the night rather than being replaced with more NREM sleep.

To complete the picture of interdependence between sleep and mood, one of the key effects of many antidepressant medications is to increase the availability of neurotransmitters such as serotonin and norepinephrine, which in turn act to suppress REM sleep. This often leads to a clinical quandary. Drugs that effectively improve mood, including such first-generation serotonin-specific reuptake inhibitors (SSRIs) as fluoxetine (Prozac) and paroxetine (Paxil), are also prone to disrupting sleep. A more recently developed antidepressant, mirtazapine (Remeron), is more specific in its effect on serotonin, as well as acting on norepinephrine. Mirtazapine is associated with less sleep disruption, although daytime sedation and weight gain may be especially problematic.

Effects on sleep and wakefulness often prove to be deciding considerations in utilizing antidepressant medication, both when insomnia is comorbid with depression and, in off-label usage, when insomnia presents alone. The sedating effects of mirtazapine as well as trazodone (Desyrel), doxepin (Sinequan), and amitriptyline (Elavil) are commonly deployed in these contexts. For depressed patients who are burdened by daytime sleepiness, the activating antidepressant bupropion (Wellbutrin) may be chosen. There are, of course, many factors guiding the choice of a particular drug or drug combination; these must be weighed in consultation with your healthcare provider.

DRUGS CAN HELP, BUT SO CAN YOU

"So," you may be thinking at this point, "I'm glad the drug companies are on it, but I thought you were offering non-drug treatments for insomnia. I'm already working with my doctor to deal with the depression; meanwhile, how do I get better sleep?"

Well, as psychologists we're glad you asked, because the interactions between depression and insomnia can be leveraged apart from recourse to polysomnographic testing or medication. These disorders not only share neurophysiological underpinnings and neurotransmitter linkages, it turns out they are both susceptible to change *when you think and act differently.*

We should not really be surprised this is so. True, over much of the twentieth century there were major disagreements over whether the mind was even a reasonable subject for study. Early in that century, strict behaviorists insisted that the mind must remain a "black box." Only what went into that box and what came out of it were open to observation, and hence to scientific inquiry. Fifty years later, when the authors of this book were undergoing graduate training, "biological psychiatry" was ascendant. "Yes, you could look into the box," this view said in essence, "but all you are going to find in there are molecules." The mind was still considered off-limits in discussions, a retrograde perspective that led nowhere.

This is clearly no longer the case. While no one has quite managed to see an idea, currently researchers are having increasing success in associating memory consolidation, puzzle solving, decision making, emotional processing—all cognitions whirling inside the black box—with observable alterations in neuronal firing rates, neurotransmitter levels, or brain structure. At this point, most practitioners are comfortable with the notion that the mysteries of the brain can be unraveled using either physical or psychological phenomena as starting points, and that the brain can be *changed* from either direction as well.

In line with this precept, there is ample evidence supporting the effectiveness of *both* psychological and pharmacological treatments for depression. The benefits of psychotherapy were originally demonstrated using psychodynamic modalities; more recent studies have focused on the effectiveness of cognitive behavioral therapy and other newer techniques. These benefits rival those of pharmacotherapy—and what is more, they are seen as at least partly additive: the combination of psychotherapy and pharmacotherapy yields better outcomes than either treatment standing alone.

Similarly, there is strong evidence for the effectiveness of *both* cognitive behavioral therapies and hypnotic medication for treatment of insomnia. We will have much to say about indications and strategies for hypnotic usage, as well as how to counter psychological dependence when trying to wean yourself off of sleeping pills, in our final chapter. Here we merely wish to emphasize that the interplay between psychology and neurophysiology, so clearly demonstrated in insomnia and depression, is, in accord with the discussion above, two-way: thoughts and actions may originate in the brain, but as they are accomplished, *they change conditions in the brain.* Therefore, they cannot help but change both your mood and your sleep. So let's turn our focus now to the dysfunctional thoughts and maladaptive behaviors that keep you from feeling and sleeping your best.

WHAT HAS DEPRESSION CHANGED ABOUT YOU?

Both mood and sleep disturbances are all-encompassing; they work against you day and night. If you struggle with the two at once, it's as if you live in a bog. Everything seems coated with gloom, sapped of vitality—your thoughts, perceptions, beliefs, and actions. To break out of this morass, you must stand ready to reconsider your most entrenched attitudes and habits—especially the ones that evolved in response to your struggles!

The first step in this process is simply to recognize what might be changed for the better. Viewed through the dark lens of depression, this preliminary task is not so simple. It is easy, given your hopelessness, to feel that *nothing* can change. You assume the dreary landscape around you to be your natural habitat; your despondent thoughts and ineffectual actions to be reflections of your true self. In fact, however, much about you *did change*, in response to years of dealing with depression and insomnia. Even allowing for genetic predispositions, you learned a lot of bad habits, and took on a lot of unhelpful beliefs, in arriving at your present predicament. In common parlance, "you are no longer yourself." Fortunately, these maladaptive lessons can be reversed.

Just a cursory listing will demonstrate the various means by which depression works its changes:

1. It reduces physical activity.
2. It curbs interests and engagement.
3. It diminishes social interaction.
4. It limits exposure to daylight.
5. It leads to unfounded beliefs, catastrophic thinking, and distortions of self-image.

Unfortunately, the broad spectrum of depression's ill effects finds a perfect match in the susceptibility of sleep to multiple influences. Let's review some of their more harmful interactions here. In the next section, we'll show you how to best counter them.

Reduced Physical Activity

The sleep/wake cycle is normally paralleled by a rest/activity cycle. There is supposed to be peak activity during the day, and limited movement, whether during brief arousals from sleep or actual awakenings, at night. Depression tends to chip away at the rest/activity cycle from both sides. During the day more hours are spent at home. And with recliners, couches, and beds at the ready, more of those at-home hours are spent at rest or napping. On the other hand, depression tends to increase activity at night, due to agitation, diurnal mood variation (with the energy and motivation to get things done finally appearing toward evening), delay of the circadian sleep phase to late hours, and outright sleep disturbance.

The upshot of all of these changes is that in depression, days tend to contain less activity, nights more activity, and both days and nights more hours in bed not sleeping. These disruptions combined can practically flatten the sleep/wake cycle.

As that cycle weakens, one hour begins to feel much like any other in terms of alertness and energy, which is to say pretty blah. By day you are too lethargic to tackle household chores, too exhausted to work in the garden. There is no way you could even think of going to the gym. When you sit down with a book or magazine you feel too befuddled to read—concentrated mental effort is out of the question. Your attention is held only intermittently by the drone of the TV. Ironically, it is then that you may drop off to sleep, when you are not intending to do so.

After such a lackluster day, by nightfall you are really feeling out of sorts. Without having accomplished much of anything, you are still somehow exhausted. You would love to be able to get a good night's sleep and start over fresh in the morning. However, that isn't happening: without a strong sleep/wake cycle, without a pent-up sleep drive borne of prolonged, engaged wakefulness, you cannot be truly sleepy. There is nothing left to pull you into slumber.

Reduced Interests and Pleasures

It will hardly be news to you that depression drains your interest in the outside world, and robs you of its pleasures. But what does giving up on guitar lessons or attending that film series have to do with your not being able to sleep? The answer lies in the diminished *quality* of your waking hours, when you are shorn of enthusiasm.

Perhaps you can still remember a time when you used to enjoy favorite activities. If so, do you recall how you used to lose yourself in them, to the point that you were not even aware of time passing? That is what is called being "in the flow." When people are fully engaged, highly motivated, and deriving pleasure from what they are doing, even sustained activity can feel almost effortless. They stay focused, on task, and alert.

That flow, along with the sense of accomplishment engendered by "peak experiences," is of course utterly lost in depression. Your progress through the day is stymied; the hours seem to unwind in slow motion. You stare at dishes rather than washing them. If you try to pick up a novel, your eyes glaze over the page. Former hobbies go unpursued. Nothing gets done, nothing is enjoyed—but you feel exhausted anyway. As we learned in the previous chapter, such blanket fatigue may lead to plenty of rest, but precious little sleep.

Reduced Social Interaction

Before modern times people generally banded together for safety to sleep—dark, quiet, and private bedrooms are a rather recent invention! Today, whether we sleep alone or not, there is still a residual sense of security brought into bed from our daytime affiliations. Young children learning to settle themselves at night are taught to rely on these bonds explicitly, assured that "mommy or daddy will be just outside." We adults are really not so grown up in this regard. Awake in the middle of the night, it remains easy enough for us to feel as if we are all alone in the world, the only ones up at that hour. This sense of alienation is only magnified if, due to depression, your day has been spent in near-solitary confinement.

The social withdrawal of depression also reduces the need to synchronize to the outside world, with a corresponding weakening in the fixed timing or *entrainment* of the circadian sleep/wake cycle. You tend to decline the invitations and duck the obligations that would require you to be away from home at a certain hour. In this, the changes wrought by depression have been abetted by technology, which now allows you to communicate with minimal typed utterances, shop from your bed, and bank with clicks, all at times of your choosing.

Regular meals are another common casualty of depression. In some cases this reflects a direct loss of appetite, one of the classic "vegetative symptoms" of the disorder. However, it may also relate to the social withdrawal and loosening of time constraints we have been discussing. Research into obesity has established that we eat not only because we are hungry but also because of external cues. That is, while sometimes we heed that growling in our stomachs, at other times we are more mindful of the clock on the wall indicating lunchtime, or the presence of others who are sitting down to a meal. Thus, in depression you may be missing or less attentive to both the internal and external cues that regulate food intake.

As a result of this dysregulation, you may do some meager snacking during the day, with sporadic meals, or outright bingeing, at night. Guts have circadian rhythms too—if you need evidence of this assertion, just try feeding your pet an hour later than usual! The clocks regulating digestive processes are weakened by haphazard food intake. This in turn deprives you of yet another means by which your sleep/wake cycle might be strengthened for better sleep.

Limited Daylight Exposure

We now turn to a discussion of two last things that have changed dramatically since your mood and sleep problems began—the light that enters your head and the thoughts that come out of it. When you are depressed, you are in the shadows, both literally and figuratively. While these changes are insubstantial in the physical sense, there are none more important to redress when it comes to getting sleepy and sleeping well.

In humans the light/dark cycle created by the Earth's rotation is the primary influence on circadian rhythms. Our eyes have specialized nonvisual receptors looking for light, in the deep blue wavelengths roughly corresponding to a clear midday sky. These receptors do not project to the occipital lobe as do others involved with color vision but rather send signals to the suprachiasmatic nucleus of the hypothalamus, the master circadian clock that regulates our core body temperature, sleep/wake cycle, and a multitude of other rhythms. From there, the signals reach the pineal gland, responsible for secreting the hormone melatonin, which in turn facilitates sleep.

So long as light of sufficient intensity enters the eye, pineal melatonin production is suppressed. As the sun sets and the daylight dims, a threshold is reached, at which point melatonin secretion begins. We certainly do not go to sleep right away when this happens. Melatonin onset occurs at dusk, while sleep typically appears four to six hours later. However, the evening buildup of melatonin is critical to getting sleepy.

Back when our ancestors spent their days hunting or gathering in the fields, retiring to huts or caves only to sleep, the physiological arrangement described above pretty much guaranteed a clear-cut light/dark cycle, and a strongly entrained rhythm of sleep and wakefulness. While various other sources of light have been available at least since the discovery of fire, Edison's demonstration of the electric lightbulb on the last day of 1879 marked the first major breach in a scheme that had served us well through eons of evolution.

Within the bat of an eye, relatively speaking, we are now all exposed to artificial light for hours after the sun has set. Millions of us also find ourselves working nights, under very bright lights, and then craving both darkness and quiet during the day, when both of these balms for sleep are in short supply.

You may not be working nights, but given your depression you might as well be, for all the natural daylight you're likely to receive on a typical day. It's fair to guess that lately you would choose to stay home over taking a long walk. While inside, you are probably not a great fan of sunshine pouring through the windows, and may in fact keep the blinds drawn. So these days (and, of course, nights!) you're more apt to be bathed in light from a computer screen than from the sun.

You may have read that light from computers and other screens can suppress melatonin, and be wondering why this light can't just serve as a substitute for sunlight. There are two main reasons why this won't work, convenient as it would be. First, direct sunlight is tremendously more intense than light produced by a screen, which leads to much stronger entrainment of circadian rhythms. Second, the fact that you can obtain your "screenlight" exposure any time you wish, with merely the flip of a switch, wreaks havoc on these rhythms. It's not simply a matter of obtaining light, *but light at a consistent time each day*, that sets up a strong circadian cycle to help you get sleepy at bedtime.

Dysfunctional Thinking in Depression and Insomnia

The most insidious change that has occurred in your struggle with mood disturbance and sleeplessness relates to how you think—about yourself, your prospects, and the world you live in. Given the interdependence of depression and insomnia, you have no doubt fallen prey at times to a vicious cycle where poor sleep and mood disturbance seemed to form a tag team, doubling up to knock you down. It's understandable that a sense of futility would take root under these circumstances. You have grown to see yourself as simply "a depressive," and "an insomniac." You are convinced that nothing will go right for you, either by day or by night.

You may even feel that, somehow, you deserve your fate. To this way of thinking, you were born with an irredeemable defect, or did something awful in the past for which you are receiving payback. You may see your sleep and mood disturbances as evidence of personal failure, or of the fact that you are just unlucky. Whatever beliefs regarding causation you have settled on, they are not only unjustified by past events but maladaptive in terms of your present functioning and future prospects—that is, they are *dysfunctional*.

Dysfunctional thinking is likely detrimental to healing of all sorts of ills. But it is especially pernicious to you, *as both broken sleep and depressed moods are directly wors-*

ened by distorted, negative thoughts. If you berate yourself day and night, your mood will inevitably darken. If you are convinced that you will not be able to sleep, you will indeed have a rough night, as the agitation and anxiety triggered by this belief are such effective barriers to sleep. If you think that failure is a foregone conclusion, you cannot possibly marshal the effort needed for success. If your mind ricochets between shortcomings and worst-case scenarios, you cannot settle into the quiet detachment sleep requires.

In these ways and more, your thinking has indeed changed for the worse, in predictable response to long battles with depression and sleeplessness. Yet all this really proves is that thinking can change—*and it can change again.* You are not forever beholden to your dysfunctional beliefs just because they currently hold sway. Now is the time for you to begin to think anew.

• • •

"You want me exercising, socializing, engaging in new interests, getting outdoors, and being more positive. If I could do all that," you might well be thinking, "I wouldn't be depressed!" We readily admit that these recommendations all require extra effort, at a time when you have very little to spare. Hopefully it has at least become clear *why* you should reconsider so much about how you think and act. Depression has changed you in many ways, and just as sledding downhill doesn't require nearly as much work as climbing back up, it will take more effort to turn these changes around. But remember, your dysfunctional beliefs and maladaptive behaviors are directly interfering with your sleep—the reason you picked up this book in the first place! And poor sleep, in turn, is exacerbating your depression. In short, you are caught in a vicious cycle.

GUARDING AGAINST FAILURE

One reason vicious cycles are so hard to break is that they build up a momentum. This can keep them spinning for quite a while, even when you're making changes for the better. It's easy to lose faith when all your extra effort doesn't seem to be paying off. You're likely to go back to your old ways, convinced that the changes you made were worthless, when in fact you were heading in the right direction.

So here's what we'll ask of you: we'd like you to make incremental, sustainable changes to nearly everything that happens in your waking hours—that is, to everything *except* your sleep. Our strategy is akin to those dieticians who aim to instill healthy eating habits in their clients while encouraging them to lose their single-minded focus on what the scale is reading. We will not be asking the impossible. We will be encouraging you to be forgiving in evaluating your progress, and to claim partial victories whenever you can. What we cannot do, however, is let you drop the ball.

"Failure is not an option," that old mantra of coaches and business leaders, may itself have bitten the dust in this new age, when tech entrepreneurs are celebrated for daring to fail before hitting pay dirt. However, in a way, that catchphrase does apply here. For when you give up on an effort, more is lost than the goal itself. Perhaps even more devastating is the effect the letdown has on what you think of yourself and your potential. Effective leaders instill confidence by *showing the way* to a goal. Anyone can set an impossibly high benchmark, but what really works is finding *the right degree of challenge* to bring out your best effort, and then pushing forward with persistence.

Let's say, for example, that you get all fired up after reading this book, and vow to be out of bed at 8 A.M., rather than your usual noon. That pledge is likely to have all the staying power of a New Year's resolution. Instead, ask yourself, what are you prepared *to achieve*, not just *try*? A concerted effort to rise by 11 A.M. or even 11:30 A.M. for the next week will be much more helpful to your cause than pulling yourself out of bed very early a couple of times in a row and then giving up out of exhaustion. In fact, even if you do stay in bed until noon one day, but get back on track the next, we will count that as a victory, not a failure.

GUARDING AGAINST SUCCESS

We've pointed out that your efforts to change are threatened by the momentum inherent in vicious cycles. That inertia poses a risk for everyone who happens to be caught in one. However, there is another reason why we have to guard especially closely against your giving up: even when things are going well, when your efforts are being met with success, *you will still be tempted to revert to your old ways*! We and a lot of other clinicians are still puzzling this out—it's a pattern that goes to the very core of depression.

The successful experiences of people who are not depressed tend to be reinforcing, in line with operant conditioning models. These experiences bring rewards, whether material or intrinsic, which in turn make it more likely that they will be repeated. People who are not depressed are also more likely to *credit themselves* following success. It's as if they make notations in some ledger of self-image: "I'm a person who *can* do this, who *enjoys* doing this, who is *effective.*"

On occasion, you too do things that bring a degree of satisfaction. The problem is that they just never seem to amount to much, let alone snowball. "Yeah, that was okay, but so what?" might sum up your prevailing attitude. You are also much more reluctant to give yourself credit when due. "It was probably a fluke," might be your thinking about something that went well. Or, "It wasn't really that good." Or, "It felt foreign to me." The effect of all this negative spin is to scuff the shine right off your success. Deep down you don't feel like it really changed anything.

The cerebral cortex, that furrowed headquarters of "higher functioning" most people picture when they think of a brain, is where these distorted thoughts, negative self-evaluations, and hopeless attitudes reside. That is why bolstering sleep regulatory mechanisms is so important for all who suffer both insomnia and depression. These mechanisms are *subcortical.* They are hard at work *underneath* the cerebral cortex, and can respond to inputs *other than thoughts.* This means that sleep regulatory mechanisms can be tapped to help you overcome your insomnia *even when you are beset by doubts.*

On the other hand, if we hope to change the ways

you act and think, we must venture right into the cortex. Here skepticism and futility abound, and opportunities for self-sabotage are rife. So we must bargain for forbearance. We promise to take your depressed circumstances into account as we make our recommendations in the coming pages. In return, we ask that you sign up for the long haul, with the understanding that even the most modest changes for the better should be retained, rather than spurned as "not working" because overall you still have depression or insomnia.

WHAT'S THE POINT OF GETTING OUT OF BED?

This is the key question on which we need to reach agreement, if you hope to make headway against your sleeplessness and depression. If you seem to be living in your bed these days, you no doubt have your reasons. It may be the refuge to which you flee because the outside world is inhospitable. It could be the cave where you hibernate, where you avoid the light of day. It may be a hideout where you give the slip to those who would pester you. It may be a shelter where you are able to deal with life in small doses, distracting yourself with phone apps. Your mattress may feel gritty and stale, but at least it always lies ready to catch you if you do nod off.

Your bed has in essence become a good place to be depressed, if not such a great place to sleep.

As you may have surmised, eventually we do want you out volunteering at your neighborhood school and swimming at the Y. *But for now we just want you out of bed.* At the absolute minimum, if it's really all you can muster, your daytime behavioral repertoire may consist solely of sitting in a chair, being depressed, and occasionally walking around outside, being depressed. Indeed, it may seem that the first steps of your insomnia treatment are going backward. Instead of resting, and perhaps falling asleep, we want you to be moving as much as possible so that there is no chance of sleep. Instead of helping you shed your struggles, we will initially be adding one more to the list—the struggle against gravity!

It's okay if while seated in your chair you wrap yourself in the same tattered blanket you were just lying under. It's okay if while on your walk you play the same candy-colored phone games that had you hooked at home—so long as you watch out for traffic, too. We are not asking you to trade in your depressive worldview just yet. We just want you to view the world with your head held upright instead of plopped down on a pillow.

Why are we keeping you from bed, the one place where you garner some comfort? It's really not to add to your misery. This one simple intervention yields benefits on many brain levels. Starting from the cortical top: As the learning theory behind stimulus control instructions emphasizes, you now associate the bed with just about everything except sleep. We need to reverse that maladaptive learning. There will also be many more opportunities for sensory and social stimulation if we can get you out in the world, which in turn promotes daytime arousal.

On subcortical levels, we need to conserve your homeostatic sleep drive, in line with sleep restriction therapy. This sleep drive is being squandered by excessive bedrest, microsleeps, and outright dozing. We also hope to increase energy expenditure by removing the support of the mattress and getting you moving instead. Last but certainly not least, by increasing daytime light exposure we will better entrain your circadian sleep/wake cycle, augment its waking portion, and, at least for some of you, directly improve your mood.

All of this, and more, is the point of your getting out of bed.

KEEP TRACK OF YOUR PROGRESS

To improve your sleep, we're asking you to make many changes in your waking life. Reducing bedrest, increasing physical exercise, getting more light exposure, regulating meals, engaging in more activities, going on outings with friends—just thinking about such a varied list of recommendations can be overwhelming, let alone actually trying to follow through on them! Moreover, we're certainly not the first clinicians to make such recommendations. There have likely been many times when you thought you were making a good faith effort to change your life, only to somehow find yourself back in the same old ruts.

What happened? Were you only going through the motions, with no real intention to change? Not necessarily. The problem may have been that daily life is complicated and full of surprises. It's hard to sustain any change in the face of the usual onslaught of last-minute errands, engine trouble, mounting paperwork, meal preparation, twisted ankles, and other demands on our attention. Most of us settled long ago on some personal triage system that deals with our most pressing issues and lets others slide, while we hope for the best. In the maelstrom of daily life, even sincere efforts to change may get lost, and any improvements rendered hard to see. This is why we urge you to track your progress. It's a lot easier to detect the "signal" of change amid the "noise" of random fluctuations in sleep and mood if consistent records are kept.

These days, of course, there is plenty of technology to assist you. There are wrist devices that quantify your daytime activity and infer your sleep patterns, alarm chimes on your phone to get you out of bed and remind you of appointments, and thousands of apps that organize your day, record your mood, monitor your food intake, promote mindfulness, and more. If you have the inclination and opportunity to use them, go ahead and indulge. The ability to record daily changes in the amount of steps you have taken is especially useful, and may warrant a moderate investment. However, even if you only keep a notebook to record your patterns, perhaps with columns devoted to minutes walked, meal times, friends visited, and some of the other criteria we have been emphasizing in this discussion, it will definitely help.

A big reason why we are so keen on having you track your progress is that it provides a tangible sign of *commitment to a goal*. Your monitor may read only 1,397 steps the first day you try it and 1,922 the next, when you thought you were going all out. Implicit in those readings, however, is another number—a goal, say, of 5,000 steps—that has thereby become more real.

Your goal also becomes more real when you tell others about it. Public declaration makes your effort a matter of record, and more difficult for you to quietly abandon. It allows you to benefit from the encouragement of others, at times when your own is in short supply. Finally, when you do reach your goal, tracking gives you clear evidence of your triumph. The little screen says 5,000, proving that it really happened. Given your tendency to diminish your accomplishments, this is not a trivial benefit!

LIGHTEN UP

Light is a natural antidepressant. This is perhaps most clearly exemplified in seasonal affective disorder, or SAD, in which the recurrence of depression is tied to changes in daylength, typically as the photoperiod shortens in the fall and is at low ebb in the winter. Seasonal depression by definition remits with the return of longer days in the spring and summer. However, it can also be treated, as well as prevented from recurring each fall, by using specially designed light boxes that emit intense light with filters in place to block harmful ultraviolet radiation. (This type of treatment is discussed more fully in chapter 6, "Are You Too Out of Sync to Sleep," since the same devices are used to treat circadian rhythm disorders.)

Following a pioneering study by Daniel Kripke in 1981,

research has pointed to a possible role for light therapy in cases of depression even when seasonal variation is not prominent. A recent meta-analysis (a statistical means of combining the outcomes of numerous research studies on a given topic to get a clearer picture of the overall results), published by Stefan Perera and colleagues in the *British Journal of Psychiatry*, evaluated twenty of the more rigorous studies in this area. While the authors rated the *quality* of the evidence they examined to be low (due to generally small sample sizes, high risk of experimental biases, and other methodological problems), they did note that the combined results do indicate a small to moderate treatment effect for light in nonseasonal depression. Subjects receiving light therapy were significantly more likely to achieve a 50 percent reduction in depressive symptoms than those in placebo conditions.

While more work may need to be done to nail down the role of light therapy in treatment for nonseasonal depression, in clinical practice it is increasingly being deployed in this context. The prominence of sleep disturbance in *your* history, persisting along with depression, convinces us that, if light does not pose special risks for you, you shouldn't wait to get more of it into your life.

These special risks include:

1. Conditions that render the eyes more vulnerable to damage from bright light, including macular degeneration and retinal dystrophies.
2. Medical disorders that increase sensitivity to light, such as porphyria and lupus, or a history of skin cancer.

3. Medications that increase sensitivity to light, including the phenothiazines, antiarrhythmic drugs such as amiodarone, and St. John's wort.
4. A history of bipolar disorder, given clinical evidence that bright light treatment can trigger manic or hypomanic episodes.

This list, of course, is not at all comprehensive; it merely serves to underscore the point that everyone who is considering light therapy, whether via a light box or natural light, should first consult with their healthcare provider to determine whether the treatment can be safely administered.

Most systematic research on light therapy in depression—seasonal or not—has administered light in the morning. In those that specifically evaluated morning vs. evening administration, response rates were greater with morning light. Indeed, clinically we see most people responding well to morning light exposure—although it has long been known that there are exceptions to this rule.

Michael Terman and colleagues, who have done much work in this area, have tied the antidepressant effect of light exposure in both seasonal and nonseasonal depression to its ability to phase advance an individual's circadian rhythms. There is an optimal window in which to obtain the light exposure, which this group has pegged between 7.5 and 9.5 hours after the onset of evening melatonin secretion. The exact timing of melatonin onset is not so easy to obtain at home. Dr. Terman has instead adapted a simple questionnaire (the Morningness-Eveningness Questionnaire, reproduced in chapter 6) to yield an estimate of when light exposure should optimally begin. A reference to a website presenting this information is included in our list of resources. In practice, relatively short sleepers who do well with about seven hours per night can begin light exposure at their normal rising time, whereas longer sleepers may have to set an alarm to rise a bit earlier to begin treatment.

The upshot of all this chronobiology is that a little personal experimentation may be in order. Most of you should be able to enjoy a stroll, or some reading under a light box, to get your mood-enhancing light in at the time suggested by Terman's group. If you opt to go outdoors, daylight, as opposed to direct sunlight, is more than sufficient on a clear day and on most cloudy days. However, on fully overcast winter mornings, the ambient daylight of about 1,000 lux (a unit of measurement, referring to light intensity on a surface) is substantially lower than the 5,000 to 10,000 lux produced by current light boxes. And of course during the winter months the sun may not even have risen at your appointed hour, necessitating use of a light box. If light treatment leads to more frequent early morning awakenings, you may have to start it thirty or sixty minutes later in the morning, reduce its duration, or, if using a light box, switch to a lower intensity or physically move the device another six inches or so away.

A relative few of you may ultimately do better with evening light. This would be most clearly indicated if you consistently experience the evening sleepiness and early awakenings characteristic of an *advanced* sleep phase, but you could also just be one of those evening light responders that seem to crop up in research studies now and then.

Finally, if it is all you can do to go outside *sometime* during the day, *whenever* you can muster the energy, and throw all the research we have been discussing to the winds—well, that's a start.

SELF-MEDICATION IN INSOMNIA AND DEPRESSION

Earlier we touched on how the choice of antidepressant medication is often influenced by a specific drug's effects on sleep and wakefulness. Of course, many people with depression turn to more everyday substances to regulate arousal level, namely alcohol and caffeine. There is a growing research literature suggesting that, for most individuals, the health benefits of moderate consumption of both alcohol and caffeine may actually outweigh the risks. Our discussion here focuses on particular downsides to relying on these substances to "treat" insomnia and its daytime consequences, in the context of depression.

Alcohol is typically consumed to hasten sleep onset, given that it may temporarily disengage us from our troubles, and is initially sedating. While a moderate amount of alcohol consumed with dinner can reasonably be part of an evening wind-down, using alcohol at bedtime to promote sleep is not a recommended practice. In addition to the general dangers of alcohol abuse and dependence, it can readily lead to a specific reliance with regard to initiating sleep.

Moreover, an alcohol-induced sleep is not restful. Unlike hypnotic medication, alcohol was not originally formulated to improve sleep, and its pharmacokinetics are all wrong for that purpose. As nightcaps are metabolized during the first hours of sleep and withdrawal sets in, the sedating effects of alcohol are in essence reversed. We suffer increased sleep fragmentation and outright awakenings, disrupting our sleep when it is supposed to be at its deepest.

Caffeine is another drug on which people with depression and insomnia often rely, in this case to battle daytime sleepiness and/or fatigue. As with alcohol, its sleep-related pitfalls stem from ready availability. There is no limit to how much caffeine you may procure—in various forms it is available on virtually every street corner—and so you may find yourself using larger quantities as you become habituated to its effects. At a certain point, you are more likely to take notice of problems with mood, focus, and lethargy when you *do not* consume your usual quota, in contrast to any perceived benefits when you do.

With regard to caffeine, again we counsel moderation. A useful strategy is to first gradually taper yourself down, over several weeks, to a "maintenance" dose of one or two cups consumed between morning and noon, and then reserve early afternoon intake for those "bad days" when you could really use invigorating. Given that the alerting effects of caffeine can linger for eight hours or more, we would advise against any caffeine consumption after midafternoon except in special cases, such as long drives, where safety is a concern.

RETHINK YOUR WAY TO SLEEP

This heading may meet with some skepticism, especially since we have seen that good sleepers rarely think much about sleep at all. Of course, they have not had the opportunity, afforded by interminable nights of insomnia, to form opinions on the subject! However, the negative thoughts about sleep occupying a central location in *your* mind are perhaps the closest thing we have to a daytime marker of insomnia. They will need to be revised or replaced if you hope to sleep well.

Earlier, we highlighted the ways in which your struggles with depression have changed the way you think. These include an increased propensity toward catastrophic thinking, self-defeating beliefs, helplessness, hopelessness, and other cognitive distortions. We are not expecting you to jettison all these maladaptive thoughts and beliefs just because we ask you to, or even because such a wholesale repudiation would, in fact, benefit both your sleep and life in general.

As those who have survived traumatic disturbances of all sorts can attest, people cannot dislodge memories, beliefs, emotional reactions, and other productions of the brain merely because they know they would be better off doing so. Like a chef hoping to adjust the flavor of a stew, we are much more capable of *adding* something to the complex mix of cognitions swirling around our minds to effect a change than removing something that shouldn't have been there in the first place.

What you'll want to add are *competing thoughts and beliefs* that cover the same mental ground, but are not quite so dire. For example, even if you believe that a worst-case scenario is inevitable, challenge yourself to come up with some plausible alternatives. If to your thinking a particular situation appears hopeless, ask yourself what would have to change to signal better prospects. Though convinced that you are utterly incapable of performing some action, imagine how someone else might fashion words of encouragement for you. Try not to let any of your long-held negative beliefs go unchallenged by some workaround, rejoinder, or reinterpretation.

The next step is to do a bit of evidence gathering to see whether one of the new alternatives actually garners more support than you would have thought. When you weigh the pros and cons, an alternative might actually make more sense than your current belief. Perhaps there are ways to empirically test the various alternatives, with some sort of informal experimentation. There are numerous specialized techniques used for such *cognitive restructuring*, the approach originated by Aaron Beck and colleagues that has become the basis of cognitive therapy. In our resource list we direct you to some sources that can get you started along this path, and of course there are many practitioners of cognitive therapy who can provide personal guidance.

Cognitive restructuring typically takes place over weeks and months rather than years, but during that time it still requires sustained effort and patience. Dysfunctional thoughts are deep-rooted, and while they continue to hold sway, your view of the world tends to be biased in ways that prop up their claims. However, just as you can pull at an invasive weed with all your might, seeming to get nowhere before it suddenly pops out of the ground, so it is that dysfunctional thoughts are sometimes surprisingly easy to displace when they've reached the limits of their support, and one last tug is applied. There can be a moment of insight, and finally, *something else* truly makes sense.

Karen, a seventy-four-year-old woman, couldn't even begin to deal with her insomnia because she showed up so late for her sessions. Karen's tardiness was due to her reliance on the bus to cross over from her home in Queens to Greenwich Village, a journey that might take an hour if all went well, trafficwise, but could just as often require two hours. It turned out that Karen had not used the subway, which would have cut the trip to about thirty minutes, for over three decades.

There are plenty of reality-based reasons to shun subway travel in New York, but Karen's chief concern was not among them. She was prone to catastrophic thinking, by day as well as by night. Years earlier, when she was still riding the subway, Karen had started to panic when the trains momentarily stopped on the tracks. Although she knew it "sounded crazy," she felt they might somehow get stuck there permanently. It didn't take much work together for Karen to recognize that it was the prospect of having a panic attack in front of dozens of strangers that was the more immediate threat. Still, the catastrophic thought of being stuck underground forever remained a catalyst for that panic.

One day, I sensed that Karen was ready to try the subway again. She had suffered through a particularly brutal traffic jam on the way to my office, arriving ten minutes before her session's close. Since it was near the end of the day, we agreed to tack on a make-up session after I had seen an intervening patient. During this session, Karen maintained her newfound resolve to ride the rails, and assented to letting me accompany her to the subway platform. But of course she started having her doubts as we made our way to the station.

While still a block or two away, I mentioned that it was actually a good thing that subways do occasionally stop on the tracks. "Why is that?" she asked, the edge sharpening in her voice. I hesitated before replying, "So they don't run into the train ahead." I forged onward, going on to explain that green, yellow, and red light signals by the side of the track let subway operators know when to go, slow down, and occasionally stop to keep a safe distance.

Karen's response was immediate. "Oh, it's just like with the buses, then. They're always slowing down, and stopping too." We both could almost hear something click in her mind with those words. Without a fuss, Karen boarded a train for a speedy, uneventful ride home. Later she commented that she had needed help from a fellow passenger to negotiate transfer to another line, but "it was no big deal."

Dysfunctional thoughts dictate our worldview, but like all tyrants, they can be toppled. The key is that *you* have to participate in the challenge. My primer on track signals was something that Karen had either heard, or surely could have surmised, beforehand. However, it was only when she permitted the explanation to resonate with her own hard experience on stalled buses—when, suitably reframed, *it emanated from her*—that Karen was finally able to board a subway train again.

Similarly, it will be up to you to rethink your views on sleep, and on yourself as a sleeper. We cannot be sure exactly what those revisions will entail. You may have to decide that, whatever happened in the past, it is safe enough for you to sleep now. You may have to accept that even though the odds of dying in your sleep are not zero, they are small enough for you to take the wager and rest your eyes. You may have to let go of your conviction that your sleep switch is broken, or that a chemical imbalance renders good sleep impossible. Whatever the case, when you are ready to see things another way, sleep will see its way to you.

CHAPTER SUMMARY

- Much evidence suggests that sleep and depression are intimately linked. Clinically, early morning awakenings have long been considered a hallmark of depression. REM sleep appears earlier in the night in those who are depressed, and is more intensely packed with rapid eye movements. Furthermore, REM sleep deprivation produces a transient antidepressant effect, while drugs that treat depression typically suppress REM sleep and alter daytime alertness. Finally, depressive mood commonly follows a circadian rhythm, with increased severity in the morning and an improved outlook in the evening.
- Despite many such two-way links, until recently insomnia was seen merely as a symptom of depression, which would resolve when mood improved. Now, sleep and mood disturbances are considered mutually interdependent conditions. Either one

can affect the other. In particular, insomnia may indeed persist after a depressive bout lifts, and when it does, the chances of a future relapse into depression increase.

- Both insomnia and depression interact with thoughts and behaviors. When you think of yourself as a poor sleeper you increase the likelihood of future sleep problems, just as you can "bring yourself down" by succumbing to negatively distorted views of your prospects. Similarly, when you just feel like hibernating at home, the resulting restrictions of physical activity, bright light exposure, and social interaction may in turn exacerbate sleep and mood disturbance.

- Given the leverage over sleep and mood wielded by your thoughts and actions, we suggest that you aim for incremental, but sustainable, changes across your waking life. This includes increasing physical activity, nurturing outside interests, engaging socially, obtaining bright light, and challenging dysfunctional beliefs. We know this is a tall order, and present detailed suggestions regarding how you might actually accomplish such changes.

- Sleep is capricious, at times seeming to bestow its rewards indiscriminately. Just as it often pays to eat more healthily and stay off the scale for a while, we suggest that, as you make modest improvements to your waking life, you not be so quick to judge them against sleep. Records and tracking devices are best used to obtain a long-term view, to prove to yourself that you are in fact progressing, even if slowly.

- Your thoughts and actions have been altered by a

long history of sleep and mood disturbance. You may interpret this to mean that by now you are stuck with who you are. On the contrary, we see the fact that you once changed in response to prior experience as proof that you *can* change. As you take in new experiences, you will have the opportunity to change again.

CHAPTER FIVE

Are You Too **Anxious** to Sleep?

Anxiety may be sleep's most wily foe. Sure, there are lots of other things that can inhibit sleep just as effectively at times. However, there is something straightforward and predictable about most of these antagonists, which can usually be counted on to provide an opening for sleep. You may just have to find the right combination of position and analgesic to bring pain down from a seven to a four, for example, and sleep's regulatory mechanisms can take over from there. A sleep phase that has drifted late can be nudged earlier according to set procedures. Although physiological hyperarousal is pretty much the antithesis of sleep, when it is finally soothed by the distraction of a captivating tale, or the relaxation of a warm bath, it's not likely to reappear out of the blue.

Anxiety, on the other hand, is not so easily laid to rest. Like a forest fire that is only apparently subdued, it maintains a store of hot embers, ready to flare up upon the smallest provocation. For those of you dealing with both anxiety and chronic insomnia, the coming of bedtime is usually all that is necessary. In this chapter we explore the different ways your anxiety is manifest, why your sleep is so vulnerable to its workings, and how you can get sleepy anyway.

STATE VS. TRAIT ANXIETY

Anxiety may be conceptualized as a *trait* or a *state*. Traits refer to stable attributes, such as predispositions in temperament, appearance, or ability. Trait models focus on the extent to which the die has been cast—by the shuffle of genes at conception, if not, as the astrologers would have it, by the alignment of heavenly bodies at birth. As many of you figured out long ago, some people tend to be more anxious by nature, just as others tend to be taller or more musically inclined.

State models, by contrast, emphasize our ever-shifting moods and thoughts as we process incoming information, contemplate the future, or delve back into memory. Yet just because states are fleeting that does not mean they are negligible. A pleasurable state may be experienced as more intense than the steady contentment reflecting a personality trait. On the other hand, even though a distressing state is just a passing cloud, in its shadow the world can look very forbidding indeed.

Trait and state models of anxiety are complementary rather than opposing. In practice, that palpable apprehension barring you from sleep is a hybrid of both types. For we all can find our place somewhere along the scale of trait anxiety, between the unflappable heroes so dear to Hollywood block-busters and those characters who take their cue from Woody Allen. Similarly, we have all experienced the onslaught of state anxiety, whether on occasion, or, if we have been con-ditioned by chronic sleeplessness, every time the sun sets. In summary, we differ in our baseline anxiety level, and also in how readily, and intensely, that anxiety surges.

IS IT OKAY TO SLEEP?

Regardless of predisposition, anxiety wells up because at some level we *feel threatened*. That the threat is typically more imaginary than real, more distant than immediate, and more exaggerated than the facts warrant, does not in the least detract from its menace. What matters most is its *internal representation*, how it looks in our mind's eye. In fact, if there is a clear and present external danger we would be speaking of *fear* rather than anxiety, and we would do well to leave our comfortable beds and run!

To fall asleep, we humans, like nearly all other animals, must deem circumstances sufficiently safe to drop our guard. We then look for a secluded, comfortable place in which to lie still. True, there are lions, raptors, and other animals at the tops of food chains that need not concern themselves with such precautions. Humans, however, rely on mental faculties to maintain dominance, faculties that are only minimally engaged during sleep.

If surprised in our slumbers, we cannot count on fleet limbs to escape a threat, let alone sharp claws or teeth to vanquish it. It is likely too late to depend on our vaunted intellect. So to really be safe, we must exercise our smarts *before* the threat appears. We have to assess risks and contingencies *before* entrusting our head to the pillow. It is no wonder so many of us are anxious nightly.

The senses we depend upon to keep our brains informed are attenuated as we drift off—but not completely. To borrow a term from electronics, they are in "sleep mode." We are less responsive to sights, sounds, touch, pain, and temperature shifts. Yet we are not in a coma. If some sensation like a jolt or a loud noise manages to get through, we can reverse sleep mode quite readily, and restore reactivity to the environment. Sometimes this abrupt transition yields a confusional state that clouds our judgment and impedes effective action. At other times we may be weighed down by "sleep inertia," a persistent grogginess that, while experienced as a dulling rather than a panic, also impairs our ability to respond.

FROM VIGILANCE TO HYPERVIGILANCE

One of the earliest findings of the modern era of sleep science described the *reticular activating system*, or RAS. The RAS is a diffuse neural network, originating in the brainstem, that integrates incoming sensory signals and determines how much of an activating impulse should be sent upward into subcortical and cortical regions—that is, how much arousal is warranted by circumstances in the outside world. For a time it was incorrectly theorized that sensory stimulation funneling through the RAS was directly responsible for wakefulness.

We know now that the sleep/wake cycle is *endogenous*, or internally generated. Our circadian clock is quite capable of organizing sleep and wakefulness in a pitch-black cave if necessary—although not, as we shall see in chapter 6, in a typical twenty-four-hour pattern. However, there is a seed of truth in the original view of the RAS: while wakefulness does not absolutely depend upon sensory signals conveyed up its pathways, it is supported by the heightened arousal produced by stimuli reckoned interesting enough to notice.

When we are anxious we tend to become *hypervigilant*. We pay more attention, and consider more things note-worthy. It's as if the RAS has lowered the bar for passing sensory input along, providing more grist for the cortical mill conducting its risk assessment. Faint shadows we would normally overlook become ominous; feeble rustlings in the night become worrisome.

THREATENING THINGS, THREATENING THOUGHTS

What kinds of threat typically give rise to sleep-disrupting anxieties? Throughout most of human history the perils were direct and unambiguous. Sleep does not come easy, for example, when one has to worry about fending off hunger, vermin, disease, or marauding invaders. Sadly, it only takes a glance at current headlines to see that for many people around the globe, these fundamental threats remain at large.

Yet even those of us who enjoy the good fortune of comfort and security still find plenty of threats to sleep. This is so because the neocortex that ballooned within the skulls of our early hominid ancestors provided a habitat where new forms of menace could lurk: our ever-resourceful brains have learned how to assemble viable threats out of *mere thoughts*.

It is true that some modern threats are really just updated versions of the old scourges. Well before hunger becomes a real issue, for example, worry over meeting monthly expenses will suffice to block sleep. Most of us are not going into actual battle tomorrow morning, but the mental preparations we make for office jousting may kindle the same activating circuitry. While a fall in social media standing is not likely to have the life-or-death consequences faced by someone ostracized from tribal society centuries ago, it taps into the same ancient need for affiliation.

Apart from such retreads, we now also grapple with totally new anxieties. These evolved along with our capacity for abstraction, and from fresh opportunities to pursue higher-order goals when our basic needs were met. The development of a moral sense, for example, gave rise to ethical concerns, and, when we have fallen short, to a whole new category of sleep inhibitors. Just as soon as we could glimpse the promise of self-fulfillment, a chasm of unfulfilled aspirations yawned wide. These are not the life-threatening dangers our forebears faced, but they are more than enough to disrupt sleep.

THE THREAT OF SLEEPLESSNESS

The above examples illustrate just how treacherous is the path we must trod nightly. Yet they do not include what is perhaps the most ubiquitous threat of all, namely, *anxiety over not being able to sleep*. Many of you are no doubt familiar with this quandary. How many times have you felt that you really had nothing to worry about, nothing to warrant such chronic sleeplessness, except well-founded concerns about being unable to sleep?

Why is the fear of sleeplessness so pervasive, and so potent? It is only recently, after all, that we have been able to cite research findings emphasizing the health risks and increased mortality associated with chronic sleeplessness, as well as with its pharmacological treatments. These findings have been trumpeted throughout mainstream media; they've probably already been added to the long list of things you worry about. No, it's likely you were anxious about sleeplessness well before having to reckon with breaking epidemiological news about its grim consequences. For the distress of insomnia is much more immediate, much more personal, than that conveyed by dry statistical analyses.

Most of you have experienced the profound loneliness of waiting out a seemingly interminable night, when it appeared as if everyone else in the world were sleeping. You

have burned with aggravation while spending hours neither fully awake nor fully asleep. You have slogged through
days with your eyes smarting, propping your head in your
palm. Perhaps most upsetting of all, you have felt the panic
that comes from being out of control. One has to be in
truly dire straits not to be able to breathe, not to be able to
drink. How can sleep, something that is ultimately just as
fundamental to well-being, be left, in essence, to chance?

ERRING ON THE SIDE OF SAFETY

One of the ways in which people deal with threatening
situations of all sorts, when feeling out of control, is by
engaging in "safety behaviors." Safety behaviors are actions
taken in the mistaken belief that they allay threats, or at
least prevent the worst from happening. For example, a
person with social anxiety might mumble behind his hand
when conversing, or stick to a prepared script of responses.
As this simple example illustrates, safety behaviors often
lead to more problems, to even less of a chance that things
will go well. They also perpetuate our anxieties, as we never
learn that challenges might be surmounted if faced squarely.

The bedtime routines you developed in response to the
anxieties of nightfall are safety behaviors. A prime example is when you take sleeping pills regularly, so as to avoid
nights "with no sleep at all." Such nightly precaution will
prevent you from ever gaining confidence that you can sleep
satisfactorily on your own. The bedtimes and rising times
you consider sacrosanct, your habit of keeping the TV on

at a certain volume, your ritual of lying wide awake in bed for hours, finally transferring to the recliner to sleep—all of these responses to insomnia are safety behaviors. They reduce anxiety in the moment, but generally increase sleeplessness in the long term.

If your sleep were fine, if you were really sleeping well in your recliner with the radio blaring, we might agree to leave well enough alone. However, the fact that you are still dealing with chronic sleep problems should raise some skepticism about your chosen strategies. They are not so protective after all, and what's more, they reinforce the notion that sleep is finicky, that everything has to be arranged just so before it will deign to arrive.

AM I ASLEEP YET?

There is one safety behavior that deserves special mention; it may be familiar to you. This is the self-assessment that begins with the question, usually voiced silently, "Am I asleep yet?" It invariably concludes with the answer, "No, I am still awake." At first glance, this would seem to be an odd example of a safety behavior, because it always ends up confirming that the feared situation—sleeplessness—is in fact present. Why would you repeatedly put yourself through this hapless exercise?

On the one hand, this puzzle may be understood by considering that the mind does not always act rationally, especially when it comes anywhere near the junction between wakefulness and sleep. As crazy as it may sound, on some level you may truly expect to find yourself asleep. However (and this is the "safety" side of the story), *you may also be fearful of losing consciousness.*

How many times have you been just at the brink of dropping off, only to find yourself inexplicably catapulted back to wakefulness? While there are physical conditions such as sleep apnea or hypnic jerks that can lead to a startle at the transition into sleep, often all it takes is your conscious mind realizing that it is perilously close to losing control of what happens next. In this context, it is the declaration "No, I am still awake" that can be seen as a safety behavior, as a reassurance that control has not in fact been lost.

Here is where the anxiety of insomnia presents a special challenge: while we are often "of two minds" when daily life induces anxiety, those two minds are still clearly *both our own.* If you feel anxiety in social situations, for example, you might wish you were able to enjoy an upcoming party, but have an even stronger urge to stay home. This ambivalence may leave you feeling agitated and miserable, but it is still *you* who is doing both the wishing *and* the avoiding.

By contrast, drifting into sleep really *does* require us to relinquish control, in the sense that we hardly recognize the mind that exists at the periphery of consciousness as our own. It's as if we must pipe aboard a harbor pilot to better handle the turbulence of the passage into sleep, handing off to a mind that can remain steady as the fog closes in. Stepping aside and hoping for the best is, of course, hardly in your anxious nature. But with practice we hope to convince you that you can do it, and that indeed, everything will turn out okay.

THREE WAYS TO SLEEP WHEN ANXIOUS

How does anyone ever fall asleep when contending with anxiety? Its physiological and psychological manifestations—its rapid heart rate, muscle tension, racing mind, and sense of foreboding—would all seem to preclude the possibility. Yet it must happen all the time, for anxiety is a very common problem, and sleeping, at least now and then, is universal. In general, there are three ways this feat is accomplished.

Exhausted Sleep

The first, falling asleep out of exhaustion, is the method you probably employ now. It can take several nights of terrible sleep in a row to get to this point. Without winding down in the least, and essentially without warning, you fall into oblivion as if falling off a cliff. Occasionally you may then be blessed with a full recovery night, which serves to remind you just how sleep is supposed to work. However, as if to bait you, your deep sleep may last only a few hours, at which point you awaken with a start, heart pounding. Now feeling totally panicked, you're not likely to get much more sleep that night, nor the following one. You're well into the next miserable cycle.

This outcome is not unexpected. When you fall asleep out of exhaustion, your anxiety has not really calmed. It just has no conscious outlet for expression, no waking state to color with its symptoms. It could wreak havoc on your dreams, or be ready to rear up again when your homeostatic sleep drive, which finally just became overwhelming, has been partly sated. In this, anxiety is similar to the hyper-arousal we discussed earlier. In both cases, the opportunity to soothe distress comes in the hours before sleep. Once you are in bed it is too late.

Medicated Sleep

The second way to get to sleep when you are anxious is to rely on medication. There are numerous options along this route; all raise general concerns that are covered more fully in our last chapter.

One pharmacologic strategy directly targets anxiety. Its objective is to promote the right frame of mind and the right bodily state—in other words, to set the stage—for sleep. These *anxiolytic* medications may be administered an hour, or even a couple of hours, prior to bedtime.

We see two advantages to this approach: First, it's asking a lot of a sleeping pill to reverse a hurtling rush of anxiety and promote sleep within, say, a half hour. And if it takes much longer than that, a new overlay of worry, this time reflecting doubts whether "this is going to work," can keep sleep at bay for hours. As you wait, the peak effectiveness of your sleeping pill may have come and gone.

Second, when anxiolytic medication is taken well before bedtime, the association between that pill and sleep is weaker than it is for a hypnotic taken soon before climbing into bed. It leaves more work for you to do in getting to sleep, but consequently, you are also more apt to give yourself some credit for the sleep you get.

As discussed in chapter 4, antidepressant medications have long been prescribed with the expectation that they would deal with any insomnia appearing with a mood disorder. While insomnia is now seen as interdependent with depression rather than merely symptomatic of it, antidepressant medications are still often seen as indicated when the clinical picture includes sleep and mood problems.

Some types of antidepressant medication are particularly useful in addressing agitation and anxiety, and may therefore be especially beneficial for you. As levels of these medications build up in the blood over a period of weeks, their benefits do not necessarily depend upon bedtime dosing. Other antidepressant medications are specifically selected for their sedating or sleep-consolidating effects, in which case they are taken before bed. Unlike anxiolytics or hypnotics, antidepressant drugs are typically administered over long terms, with courses of a year or more not uncommon.

Finally, hypnotic medications can be used to induce sleep directly, even when insomnia is associated with anxiety. Working within neurotransmitter and peptide systems that promote sleep, their effect can be likened to an artificial increase in the homeostatic sleep drive. They do not so much remove anxiety as overlay it with sleep. Moreover, the mere knowledge that you are taking a *sleeping* pill provides another important mechanism of action. It yields the comforting sense that you are covered, that sleep is out of your hands. Consequently, you won't be sabotaging your sleep tonight!

In recent years the well-documented risks of these medications have been more widely publicized, and your physician may be reluctant to prescribe more than a short-term supply. What is not useful in such cases is to turn to wholesale use of over-the-counter preparations to counter your anxiety.

Diphenhydramine (Benadryl) is available, for example, in every drugstore. Apart from potential issues of memory impairment, diphenhydramine has an extra-long half-life, and is notorious for producing morning hangover effects. Melatonin is another sleep aid, readily obtained at vitamin stores. Perhaps because it is touted as natural, melatonin is often administered either in doses that are too large or too late within the sleep period. People think of it as a "sleep lozenge," to be taken as needed. However, large doses can cause significant daytime deficits. Moreover, because of the special role it plays in the timing of circadian rhythms, using melatonin to get a little extra sleep in the morning can actually make it more difficult for you to fall asleep on following nights.

While our focus as psychologists is on the nonpharmacological treatment of insomnia, we believe that there are some contexts in which sleeping pills represent a reasonable treatment option, given that they have been specifically formulated to aid sleep and clear out by sunrise. In your case, this might include the looming presence of a major, if time-limited, source of anxiety. If public speaking sends shivers down your spine, for example, but you must nonetheless prepare to address a large group a week from Thursday, you might weigh the pros and cons of obtaining a brief prescription with your healthcare provider. Yes, there are effective behavioral programs to alleviate fear of public speaking and many other phobias, but now might not be the time to start one. Even so, you are not exempted from adopting more appropriate sleep/wake practices, so as to better help your medication help you.

Becalmed Sleep

The third—and to our mind the most desirable—way to fall asleep when anxious is to first dial back your anxiety, by behaving and thinking differently *before bedtime.* To choose this path you must stop chasing sleep, and, strange as it may seem, cultivate a sense of detachment regarding the whole enterprise. Your goal, at least in the interim, should be *relaxed wakefulness* during the evening hours. Believe it or not, you can get practiced at letting yourself approach, but not pass through, the threshold of sleep. Tranquil detachment also happens to be the perfect perch from which to fall asleep once you do go to bed, but you'll want to savor it for its own sake.

You need not transform yourself into some unrecognizable, laid-back slacker to become a better sleeper. All day long you are free to charge ahead, sweat the details, and yes, even indulge in your trademark worrying. By the way, your mental gymnastics should not preclude physical exercise as well, scheduled any time up until about four hours before bedtime, since this can be a great way to dissipate anxious energy as well as extra calories.

The last couple of hours before bed, however, should have a different feel. From midevening on, no striving is allowed, no pursuit of either life goals or of sleep. You need time to construct a nightly bulwark against the swells of your anxiety by losing yourself (along with your worries) in a book, conversation, music, handicrafts, a movie, or other diversion. You may also wish to soothe your tensions with a warm bath, a massage, or some herbal tea. When you finally climb into bed, *you should already be accustomed to stillness.* Hopefully you will fall into reverie lasting fifteen or twenty minutes, for that is how long is usually required to fall asleep when conditions are right. If you have reached the proper frame of mind, however, you won't be thinking about time at all.

Why should all these soothing words be so hard to put into practice? Well, for one thing, it only takes a second or two for your nascent calm to be shattered by some stray intrusive thought, so fifteen to twenty minutes can seem an eternity. If you are able to cull them out and maintain a pleasant drift in your thoughts, great. But if you find yourself only growing more frustrated, a specialized intervention may be required. Let's take a look at how some treatments selected from the list reviewed in chapter 1 can be particularly useful for getting you, despite all your anxiety, to sleep.

DON'T TAKE YOUR ANXIETY TO BED

"Stimulus control instructions" sounds scary enough; what it asks of you—to get out of bed in the middle of the night when you cannot sleep—probably seems downright onerous. Many anxious patients decide it's not for them, which they then confirm with a few attempts that "don't work."

Here's why you should not write off stimulus control so quickly: *It was formulated expressly to remove anxiety from your bed.*

It does so in theory, as you no longer pair the anxiety and frustration of being unable to sleep with your bed, so that the association between the furniture and the distress begins to weaken. And it does so in practice, as you escape the dark chamber where you have already spent so many agonizing hours awaiting sleep, while in the throes of yet another failed attempt, to repair instead to a comfy armchair.

"So what," you may be thinking, "now I'll just be anxious in the chair, with even less of a chance to sleep!" We understand that being up in the middle of the night is not pleasant, period—and that just moving from one room to another can't be expected to change your mood. You'll have to calm down and regain your composure some other way. However, there is still value in changing venues. At this point you have a much better chance of learning how to settle yourself in an armchair, with a book, magazine, or music to distract you, than in your rumpled bed, where your only options are to succeed or fail at sleep.

Another major benefit of stimulus control, given your anticipatory anxiety about being unable to sleep, is that once you have gotten out of bed, you are no longer even trying. The helpless, out-of-control feelings that have infused your experience of insomnia are, at a stroke, reframed. Just a few minutes ago, there you were, tossing about in bed, with only your mocking, dysfunctional thoughts for company. Now, as you seat yourself comfortably, turn on some music, or turn the page, you are invited to share in *some-*

one else's experience. You have entered a new world, where you can register as a guest for twenty or thirty minutes. In this foreign land, there is no place for your unpaid bills, your spat with a colleague, your health concerns, and all the other personal issues that were so recently upsetting. Unencumbered, your mind can finally relax. It will then grow tired of the visit, and be ready for sleep.

MEDITATION

Adherents of mindfulness and other meditative practices learn a discipline that, in addition to offering many benefits for waking life, can pave the way for sleep to make its nightly appearance. Meditation is especially beneficial when sleep is inhibited by anxiety because it promotes *intention* in our inner lives: instead of merely reacting to outside influences, or being pulled helplessly along well-worn internal paths of worry, we make a conscious decision to focus on a mantra, experience the present moment, or allow ourselves to drift along an unfolding meditative scenario. As we put this intention into practice, we change the cognitive balance.

These simple acts, though playing out in the mind, still represent a concrete demonstration of purpose, every bit as much as choosing to walk a mile does. In fact, the mental venue may even prove more fortifying for you than a gym track. For when insomnia is raging, it is often your psychological, more than physical, stability that is undermined.

The soothing effects of mindfulness linger beyond the

relatively short time actually spent meditating. Its practice promotes equanimity across all your waking hours, which in turn should ease the eventual transition to sleep. Moreover, mindfulness imparts tools to which you can resort when that transition proves rocky. You can learn to stay in the present moment, so that the mistakes of the past and the uncertainties of the future loosen their grip on your pillowed head. And you can learn to string such moments together, to create the fifteen- or twenty-minute respite from worry that will render you ready for sleep.

SLEEP RESTRICTION THERAPY

We have noted that sleep restriction therapy is usually well tolerated in those whose insomnia is associated with hyperarousal, as the "side effect" of daytime sleepiness produced by this treatment seems to counter elevated arousal. The same observation holds for anxiety: Your edginess and tension, which nightly prevent you from getting sleepy, may be blunted by increasing your homeostatic sleep drive through sleep restriction.

Strange as it sounds, you may also derive a certain reassurance from experiencing moderate daytime sleepiness. As you are well aware, one of the quizzical characteristics of your insomnia is that oftentimes you don't feel sleepy during the day, even when you've slept poorly at night. This experience may lead you to question whether your "sleep is broken." Eliciting sleepiness directly, via adherence to sleep restriction treatment, confirms that the brain mechanisms responsible for sleep are indeed still in working order. Of course, getting that sleepiness to appear on cue, at the end of the evening rather than the middle of the day, remains a challenge. Still, at least there is now something for you to work with.

We spoke earlier of how sleep restriction therapy makes sleep boring. By increasing sleep consolidation while limiting time in bed, it precludes long "recovery sleeps," but also avoids total washouts. So-so sleep becomes the norm, which is actually just what you need, as this lack of variability reduces anticipatory anxiety about what the night will bring. You may still wonder how you'll ever make it to bedtime or pull yourself out of bed so early in the morning. *But those worries are not about sleep itself.* And the less you worry or even think about sleep, the better.

CAN'T READ, CAN'T SLEEP

Reading makes most people sleepy. It seems to do so more reliably than other sedentary activities, even more than just sitting quietly. For this reason, reading is usually the first choice when it comes to filling a buffer period before bed. As noted in our discussion of stimulus control instructions, one reason reading is so soporific is that it immerses us in another time and place, distracting us from our own real-world concerns.

There are of course other kinds of immersive experience, for example, movies and video games, which are much less likely to bring on sleepiness. Clearly, absorption in another world is not necessarily calming. The type of response required by a given activity appears to be critical: When stimulation is delivered wholesale, when we are called upon to react perceptually and motorically to a full barrage of information that starts to mimic reality, sleep is deferred. Perhaps such experiences are too much like waking life.

This brings up a second reason why reading makes us sleepy: It is effortful. We have to construct for ourselves the alternate world that will serve as our diversion, essentially piece by piece. We have to build that fourteenth-century Scottish castle and discern the intrigue brewing within its stone walls, enter that 1920s speakeasy and ride out the adventures of our narrator, all using just a couple dozen text symbols. Meanwhile, most of your visual field is still taking in your living room, and your ears can still hear the refrigerator cycle in the kitchen. In other words, the printed page doesn't do nearly as much heavy lifting to transport you to another world as does, say, your large-screen TV. It relies on your mind instead. This can be mentally fatiguing in a way that pulls mightily for sleep.

However, many of you cannot rely on reading to get sleepy, because you have nearly as hard a time settling into a book as into sleep. You get sidetracked or agitated within a few pages. Instead, you find yourself attracted to more active diversions. For example, clicking through an endless chain of internet links, or even fighting a virtual desert battle on a large screen, is somehow calming, even if these forays are not likely to lead to sleep.

We see your difficulties reading as linked to your difficulties sleeping. There is something about being able to tolerate partial removal from the "real" world, of having to dwell for a while inside your mind's half-formed constructions, that binds the two. Note that we do not here wish to take anything away from video gaming, and are not promoting reading as "better for you." There is no doubt that being an accomplished gamer requires substantial skill, as well as cognitive effort. It's just that that effort is more likely to trigger hyperarousal than sleepiness.

The active effort of reading, even for those who are able to sustain it, of course ceases as soon as the lights are dimmed. If you can manage to linger a few more minutes in the fourteenth century once the book is closed, or, if books are not your thing, in a reverie of your own devising, you just may fall asleep. However, as you well know, a mental vacuum can open up within seconds, into which all kinds of anxiety-inducing cognitions are eager to rush. Clearly, another tactic would be helpful here. We have found that sometimes all it takes to keep anxious thoughts at bay is a song.

WHEN LULLABIES FAIL, LEARN A NEW SONG

Recently we have begun to explore how the kind of active effort that leads to mental fatigue while reading might be fostered in bed, in the dark, with your eyes closed. Of course, many such strategies have already been proposed, most famously using a long line of numbered sheep. Nowadays people will typically listen to music, relaxation tapes, or audiobooks while in bed. Certainly the effectiveness of being read to at bedtime has a long pedigree. Nonetheless, instead of soothing you would-be sleepers with a bedtime story or lullaby, we are asking you to take on a heavier cognitive load. Specifically, we suggest that you learn the lyrics to a song.

Pick a tune that is easily hummed, but with a lot of complicated lyrics shoehorned into the melody. Reaching way back, show tunes from the Gershwins or Cole Porter fit the bill nicely. Those in our age cohort may appreciate that Bob Dylan represents a nearly inexhaustible resource in this regard. However, we will leave everyone to their own devices as far as selection. It helps if you are motivated to learn the lyrics because you really like the song! You are allowed to listen to it just once in the evening, before your buffer period.

When you first get in bed, just close your eyes and rest. If your thoughts are drifting along peacefully, we do not suggest intervening at all. However, if your mind starts to race, or unsettling thoughts begin to intrude, your only recourse is to try your best to reconstruct the lyrics to your chosen song. There are to be no headphones in bed, and no "cheating" by listening to the tune again.

It turns out that this activity is mildly pleasant at the outset, but after a while it becomes mildly annoying. The first words in a stanza and the repeating chorus are likely to be nailed early on, but the place of a lot of the other lyrics will have to be filled in with humming. Go back to the beginning and give it another try. A good tune should be catchy enough to easily drown out other contending thoughts, so you can stay with it for five minutes, maybe even ten minutes or more. After that, you will no doubt hit a wall in terms of lyric reconstruction.

Here is where the second part of the intervention comes in: you are allowed to rest your mind whenever you feel the need after your first run-through, to "put it in park," or resume an easy drift. After all, you're probably not going to drop off into sleep midlyric. However, if you find yourself starting to rev up, anticipating tomorrow's big presentation, regretting that last text you sent, or mentally sorting through your bills, you must stop what you're thinking and get yourself, once again, "tangled up in blue."

CHAPTER SUMMARY

- We all differ in our baseline level of anxiety, known as *trait anxiety*, and also in how susceptible we are to surges of short-lived *state anxiety*. Because anxiety can flare up so quickly and unexpectedly, it poses a special challenge to sleep.

- Humans, like most animals, must judge circumstances sufficiently safe to sleep. However, we are not particularly fleet of foot, sharp-toothed, or well-camouflaged, so we have to rely on our intellect for security—knowing full well that our brains will be in "sleep mode" once we drift off. This prompts us to be hypervigilant to any potential threats as bedtime approaches.

- Primordial threats to sleep were mainly external, such as adverse weather, predators, or vermin. As the human brain evolved, such threats could be internally represented as anxious thoughts, which even as they grew more abstract, proved just as adept at disrupting sleep.

- We engage in "safety behaviors" to avoid facing threatening situations directly. Safety behaviors prevent us from learning more effective ways to counter those threats. Chronic insomnia gives rise to many safety behaviors, from pillow arrangements to drug regimens, that may ease the threat of sleeplessness one night while maintaining our vulnerability the next.

- When anxious, you can eventually get to sleep in one of three ways: through exhaustion, medication, or by first attaining a measure of calm. The first two often yield a few hours of sleep, which, after paying off the worst of your "sleep debt," are followed by worry-filled awakenings. Finding repose before bedtime, by contrast, prepares the way for sound sleep later at night.

- Stimulus control instructions train you to avoid making anxiety your bed partner. The timeouts for reading or listening that it prescribes are not generic interventions; they immerse you in someone else's world for a while, where your own anxieties have no place. We see reading, especially, as involving a combination of stillness and effort that primes for sleep.

- Mindfulness-based practices can offer major benefits when anxiety inhibits sleep. By unyoking us from our worries and fostering appreciation of the present moment, they render waking hours more conducive to sleep. As mindfulness skills are honed throughout the day, they become increasingly ready to counter mind-racing and intrusive thoughts at night.

- The mere thought of sleep restriction therapy can induce worry. Yet the sleepiness it generates, by increasing the sleep drive, may be better tolerated in those with chronic anxiety—who often stand more than ready to trade in their nervous exhaustion. Sleepiness is in fact sometimes even welcomed, as proof that sleep mechanisms are not totally broken.

CHAPTER SIX

———

Are You Too **Out of Sync** to Sleep?

Sometimes the problem is not how but *when* you sleep. Most people sleep best at night, without making any particular effort to do so. However, not everyone sleeps at hours that jibe well with the Earth's light/dark cycle. Some tend to slumber early in the evening, only to wake up when it is pitch black outside. Others are wide awake all night, finally falling asleep after the sun has risen. To get a sense of just how out of sync you are, you may wish to take the Morningness-Eveningness Questionnaire, first devised by James Horne and Olov Östberg in 1976 and still widely used today.

Morningness-Eveningness Questionnaire (MEQ)

Please read each question very carefully before answering. Please answer each question as honestly as possible. Answer ALL questions. Each question should be answered independently of others. Do NOT go back and check your answers.

1. **What time would you get up if you were entirely free to plan your day?**

5:00–6:30 A.M.	5
6:30–7:45 A.M.	4
7:45–9:45 A.M.	3
9:45–11:00 A.M.	2
11:00 A.M.–noon	1
Noon–5:00 P.M.	0

2. **What time would you go to bed if you were entirely free to plan your evening?**

8:00–9:00 P.M.	5
9:00–10:15 P.M.	4
10:15 P.M.–12:30 A.M.	3
12:30–1:45 A.M.	2
1:45–3:00 A.M.	1
3:00–8:00 A.M.	0

3. **If there is a specific time at which you have to get up in the morning, to what extent do you depend on being woken up by an alarm clock?**

Not at all dependent	4
Slightly dependent	3
Fairly dependent	2
Very dependent	1

4. **How easy do you find it to get up in the morning (when you are not woken up unexpectedly)?**

Not at all easy	I
Not very easy	2
Fairly easy	3
Very easy	4

5. **How alert do you feel during the first half hour after you wake up in the morning?**

Not at all alert	I
Slightly alert	2
Fairly alert	3
Very alert	4

6. **How hungry do you feel during the first half hour after you wake up in the morning?**

Not at all hungry	I
Slightly hungry	2
Fairly hungry	3
Very hungry	4

7. **During the first half hour after you wake up in the morning, how tired do you feel?**

Very tired	I
Fairly tired	2
Fairly refreshed	3
Very refreshed	4

8. **If you have no commitments the next day, what time would you go to bed compared to your usual bedtime?**

Seldom or never later	4
Less than one hour later	3
One to two hours later	2
More than two hours later	I

9. You have decided to engage in some physical exercise. A friend suggests that you do this for one hour twice a week, and the best time for him is between 7:00 and 8:00 A.M. Bearing in mind nothing but your own internal "clock," how do you think you would perform?

Would be in good form	4
Would be in reasonable form	3
Would find it difficult	2
Would find it very difficult	1

10. At what time of day do you feel you become tired as a result of need for sleep?

8:00–9:00 P.M.	5
9:00–10:15 P.M.	4
10:15 P.M.–12:45 A.M.	3
12:45–2:00 A.M.	2
2:00–3:00 A.M.	1

11. You want to be at your peak performance for a test that you know is going to be mentally exhausting and will last for two hours. You are entirely free to plan your day. Considering only your own internal "clock," which ONE of the four testing times would you choose?

8:00–10:00 A.M.	4
11:00 A.M.–1:00 P.M.	3
3:00–5:00 P.M.	2
7:00–9:00 P.M.	1

12. If you got into bed at 11:00 P.M., how tired would you be?

Not at all tired	1
A little tired	2
Fairly tired	3
Very tired	4

13. For some reason you have gone to bed several hours later than usual, but there is no need to get up at any particular time the next morning. Which ONE of the following are you most likely to do?

Will wake up at usual time but will NOT fall back asleep	4
Will wake up at usual time and will doze thereafter	3
Will wake up at usual time but will fall asleep again	2
Will NOT wake up until later than usual	1

14. One night you have to remain awake between 4:00 and 6:00 A.M. in order to carry out a night watch. You have no commitments the next day. Which ONE of the alternatives will suit you best?

Would NOT go to bed until watch was over	1
Would take a nap before and sleep after	2
Would take a good sleep before and nap after	3
Would sleep only before watch	4

15. You have to do two hours of hard physical work. You are entirely free to plan your day and considering only your own internal "clock," which ONE of the following times would you choose?

8:00–10:00 A.M.	4
11:00 A.M.–1:00 P.M.	3
3:00–5:00 P.M.	2
7:00–9:00 P.M.	1

16. You have decided to engage in hard physical exercise. A friend suggests that you do this for one hour twice a week, and the best time for him is between 10:00 and 11:00 P.M. Bearing in mind nothing else but your own internal "clock," how well do you think you would perform?

Would be in good form	1
Would be in reasonable form	2

Would find it difficult   3

Would find it very difficult   4

17. Suppose that you can choose your own work hours. Assume that you worked a FIVE-hour day (including breaks) and that your job was interesting and paid by results. At approximately what time would you choose to begin?

Five hours starting between 4:00 A.M. and 8:00 A.M.   5

Five hours starting between 8:00 A.M. and 9:00 A.M.   4

Five hours starting between 9:00 A.M. and 2:00 P.M.   3

Five hours starting between 2:00 P.M. and 5:00 P.M.   2

Five hours starting between 5:00 P.M. and 4:00 A.M.   1

18. At what time of the day do you think that you reach your "feeling best" peak?

5:00–8:00 A.M.   5

8:00–10:00 A.M.   4

10:00 A.M.–5:00 P.M.   3

5:00–10:00 P.M.   2

10:00 P.M.–5:00 A.M.   1

19. One hears about "morning" and "evening" types of people. Which ONE of these types do you consider yourself to be?

Definitely a "morning" type   6

Rather more a "morning" than an "evening" type   4

Rather more an "evening" than a "morning" type   2

Definitely an "evening" type   0

James Horne and Olov Östberg. 1976. "A Self-Assessment Questionnaire to Determine Morningness-Eveningness in Human Circadian Rhythms." *International Journal of Chronobiology* 4 (2): 97–100. Used by permission.

Add up the scores on the nineteen questions of the MEQ to yield your total score, which can range between 16 and 86 points. If the total score is 41 or below, you are a clear "evening type." A total score of 59 or above indicates that you are a clear "morning type." Finally, if your score ranges between 42 and 58, you are an "intermediate type."

The notion that some people are morning larks while others are night owls has a venerable history. The figurative usage of "night owl," as someone who is active at night, has been traced back at least as far as Shakespeare. However, it is only in recent decades, through work in chronobiology and genetics, that the inborn mechanisms behind the morning lark's propensity to fall asleep early and the night owl's habit of staying up late are beginning to be understood.

It turns out that each of us has a master clock in our brain, more formally known as the *suprachiasmatic nucleus*, or SCN. The SCN is a pulsing cluster of neurons that sets the pace for a multitude of other internal clocks, conferring on each of us an array of *circadian rhythms*, or cycles with a period length of about twenty-four hours. The SCN regulates core body temperature, hormone release, and much else of our physiology, down to processes that take place on a cellular level.

What does a circadian rhythm look like? Suppose you measured your core body temperature every fifteen minutes for an entire week, day and night, and plotted the measurements on a graph. The resulting curve would resemble seven rolling waves as your temperature rose and fell. The time interval from one wave crest to the next would be very close to twenty-four hours.

So far, we're all the same in this. However, if on

your chart you then marked down your local clock time under the series of waves, differences would appear. For most people, each temperature crest would occur in the midevening, say, around 8:30 P.M. However, for some of you the peak might come several hours earlier, while for others it could be near midnight. The peaks and troughs of your circadian core temperature cycle, along with those of other circadian rhythms, determines when *you* are able to get your best sleep, as measured by the clock on the wall. This external clock is, of course, just a stand-in for the Earth's rotation and the light/dark cycle it produces.

In this chapter we describe chronotypes, the disorders that can arise from them, and their treatment. If our scenarios are tilted toward the night owls, it is not only because this pattern is more prevalent; it also reflects the more public consequences of sleeping late. If you are in danger of losing your job due to morning tardiness, or of being expelled from school, you are hardly alone. You should push back against the notion that your attendance problem can simply be chalked up to laziness or a lack of motivation. There is now an extensive scientific literature that establishes your chronotype as a factor warranting consideration. Let's explore what lies behind your *circadian rhythm disturbance*, and most importantly, what you can do about it.

LIVING WITH WAYWARD CLOCKS

A key finding of sleep science is that only a very few of us possess an internal clock with a period of almost exactly twenty-four hours, such that our preferred day length would perfectly match the spin of the Earth. Our SCN clocks run either too slow or too fast. Their timing can be off from a few minutes to about an hour, every cycle. This is the case even though the rhythms that they regulate, as with the waves of temperature fluctuations described above, remain synchronized or *entrained* to the wall clock. How does a faulty internal clock produce a twenty-four-hour rhythm?

The average circadian clock runs just a bit slow, with a natural period length near 24.2 hours. To stay "on time" (and thereby yield a 24-hour rhythm), it must be advanced ten or so minutes once a day, the way one might advance the hands of an antique clock that is also slow. There are numerous ways to shift the SCN; as we shall soon learn, properly timed light exposure and melatonin adminstration are the most effective. However, just as correcting the time on an antique clock does not prevent it from lagging again, resetting a circadian clock will not change how accurately it runs going forward. We can't repair the SCN the way a watchmaker might adjust a timing mechanism.

Over thirty-five years ago Charles Czeisler surmised that individual differences in the intrinsic period length of the SCN might be responsible for the existence of night owls and morning larks. Gathering evidence to back up this hypothesis has proven difficult, in part due to the laborious experimental protocols required. However, as the results trickle in they do appear to confirm Dr. Czeisler's view. The situation is a bit complicated, because differences in SCN period length appear to influence how early or late people choose to sleep as measured by their *internal clocks*, as well as by the clock on the wall. For our purposes, it's enough to know that out in the world, fast clocks seem to yield morning larks, and slow clocks night owls.

Age also appears to affect the timing of our sleep schedules. Young adults as a group are more likely to be night owls, for reasons beyond their fondness for late-night socializing, while the elderly are more likely to sleep and wake on an early schedule. For most people the drift is manageable and easy enough to reverse. It is only when the timing of sleep becomes distressing, and interferes with life activities, that we speak of *Circadian Rhythm Sleep Disorder*, of the advanced or delayed type.

Internal clocks that run extra slow, characteristic of night owls, are quite difficult to reset. You may have noticed that when the social costs of sleeping late are temporarily removed—for example, during a week of vacation—not only do you quickly revert to a very late bedtime, your sleep also starts to appear *progressively* later. Each night, for example, you may go to sleep about half an hour later than the previous night. You are "free running," that is, living according to your SCN's intrinsic (in this case, 24.5-hour) period. At that rate, it doesn't take long before your sleep phase has shifted so late that you cannot sleep until morning.

When your sleep is that delayed, you may have hit upon the strategy of just staying awake the entire day to get back on an early schedule. Such prolonged wakefulness may indeed yield you a stint of nighttime sleep, through the sheer accumulation of homeostatic sleep drive. However, this approach works well for relatively few night owls. The problem is that your internal clock is not reset by one-shot sleep deprivation. You may achieve a decent recovery sleep, but are still likely to feel out of sorts the next day. Sleep may then appear in an irregular pattern for a while, with stints of varying length occurring both day and night, before reconstituting on a late schedule again.

IS IT YOU, OR YOUR CLOCK?

That you occasionally "apply the brakes" to your shifting sleep phase, while easing off and letting your sleep drift at other times, may be cited as proof by your boss or school principal that your late arrivals reflect a choice. "It's hard for lots of people to get up in the morning," they may chide, "but most just do it when they have to." If only you would pull yourself together for a week or two, according to this line of reasoning, you could get yourself back on track and rejoin the schedule of your peers. A less judgmental variant of this attitude is offered by many healthcare providers, who prescribe a few weeks' course of hypnotic medication to be taken at the desired bedtime, again in the hopes of stabilizing sleep on an earlier schedule.

We have been clinicians long enough to know that motivational factors cannot be summarily dismissed when a teenager is in danger of being held back a year, or an employee is about to lose a job, because of excessive tardiness and absenteeism. There are also obvious social and cultural factors at work, such as online communities engaged in heated discussions through the night, or friends who expect responses to their texts no matter what the hour. Still, when asked by administrators whether "this is really biological or not," whether our patient could be on time if he or she really wanted to, we may have to give the unsatisfying response that *both* genetic and motivational factors are at work.

The situation is analogous, we might explain, to swimming against a river's current. It can usually be done for a while. Just how long depends, of course, on the swimmer's skills, strength, and, it is true, motivation, but also on the speed of the current. Some people, we emphasize, have sleep that is more markedly prone to drift than others'. They are in effect sleeping against a stronger current, *and they were born that way*. People saddled with wayward internal clocks can eventually become demoralized or disaffected from years of fruitless effort to keep to a so-called normal sleep schedule. By the time they come to clinical attention, they may well have decided to just "go with the flow." However, just because low mood and low motivation may be plainly read on the face of a dispirited teenager, while the workings of the circadian clock are hidden in his hypothalamus, that does not mean biological factors are absent.

It should be added here that the totally blind, who are not susceptible to the entraining effect of daylight, are often completely unable to halt the free running of their internal clocks. They have a non-twenty-four-hour sleep disorder; that is, their sleep shifts around the clock continually—not just during vacations as alluded to above. Fortunately, sleep in both the sighted and the blind can also be entrained by timed administration of the hormone melatonin or related substances. This has become the treatment of choice in cases of non-twenty-four-hour sleep disorder.

WHAT DOES THE CLOCK REALLY TIME?

While the concept of circadian rhythms and the notion of a "biological clock" has gained currency in the general population, there remains a lot of confusion surrounding its workings. It certainly does not "time" sleep in a manner analogous to coffee brewers or video recorders programmed to precisely turn on and off. You may generally find it easiest to sleep between 2 A.M. and 10 A.M., but even so you will not fall asleep in midsentence when the clock on the wall (or the one in your brain) strikes two. Furthermore, we're sure you can remember many times when you were snug in bed at 2 A.M. only to find yourself unable to sleep for hours!

These reflections should make it clear that the SCN ticking away in our hypothalamus does not actually put us to sleep. What it *does* do is regulate the appearance, every twenty-four hours, of our *best opportunity* for sleep. If we manage to fall asleep just as this window is opening, we are most likely to stay asleep for an adequate length of time, and with sufficient depth, to function at our best during waking hours. The circadian clock regulates many physiological rhythms to accomplish this feat, orchestrating their arrangement within our bodies the way a conductor brings up the woodwinds and tamps down the brass to achieve a particular musical effect. The key players in this ensemble are the temperature, melatonin, and cortisol rhythms.

The Circadian Temperature Rhythm

Every twenty-four hours, our core body temperature,

which we highlighted at the start of this chapter as an exemplary circadian rhythm, rises and falls about one degree Celsius. That may not sound like much, but in fact this slight fluctuation makes all the difference in terms of arousal. When the temperature cycle is near its peak we are very alert, while at its trough we are minimally alert. The circadian temperature rhythm is in fact so central to sleep and wakefulness that it often serves as a proxy for the clock itself. In *The Insomnia Answer* we assumed as much when we spoke of the circadian clock, manifested by the core body temperature cycle, as regulating the "alerting force."

We generally turn in a few hours after the core temperature rhythm has peaked, but still well before it reaches its low point. For example, if our temperature peak occurs shortly after 8 P.M., we may be ready for sleep around 11 P.M. It might seem counterintuitive that we do not wait until the circadian temperature rhythm is at its lowest before going to sleep. However, upon reflection this does make sense: if we did, we would be getting to sleep just as alertness was on the rise! We maintain sleep best while our core body temperature is falling, and as it bottoms out. As it rises, we have an easier time rising from bed.

From the foregoing it should become clear that the *timing* of your circadian temperature peak is a key determinant of how likely, at any given hour, you can successfully fall asleep. In you night owls, that temperature peak may be delayed several hours. If, in anticipation of an early start for work or school, you "try to get in a full night" and retire around 11 P.M., you will end up attempting to sleep at the hardest possible time to do so! That is why so many of you end up tossing and turning for hours.

The Melatonin and Cortisol Rhythms

Circadian rhythms in the levels of the hormones melatonin and cortisol are also critical to how well we sleep. Melatonin, produced by the pineal gland, situated between the two cerebral hemispheres of the brain, is the sleep/wake cycle's link to the outside world. When the sun is nearly down to the horizon, the pineal gland begins to secrete melatonin. We do not then fall right off to sleep, of course. Instead, the secretion and buildup of melatonin sets off a cascade of thermoregulatory and other neurophysiological changes that prepare the way for sleep several hours later.

In contrast to the soporific effects of endogenous melatonin, the secretion of cortisol by the adrenal glands is activating. After all, this is the hormone that surges to sustain effort in times of emergency, or when under chronic stress. Under normal conditions the circadian rise of cortisol levels as morning approaches helps to rouse our bodies from slumber. However, as with the core body temperature and melatonin rhythms, those of you with sleep/ wake phase disorders are also dealing with displacements in the peak of your cortisol rhythm. This peak appears late in those with a delayed sleep phase pattern, too late to be of service in helping you heed that early alarm.

LIFE OUT OF SYNC

It would be truly surprising if the only consequence of all the circadian rhythms shifted inside of you happened to be a change in bedtime. And indeed that is not the case. Practically every facet of your daytime functioning reflects these shifts as well. They affect your mood, the best time to get work done, your appetite, when you feel like socializing, and when you are likely to be exposed to light. These are not just minor changes that may be expected to fall into line once the "underlying problem" is addressed. They in fact can prevent that problem from ever getting resolved.

Let's track these consequences of a delayed sleep phase across the day, to illustrate how they keep you on a late pattern. Perhaps the most obvious consequence of falling asleep late, and setting an early alarm, is that you don't want to get out of bed when the alarm rings. In fact, many of you do not even hear your alarm, because you are still in deep sleep, with a high threshold for arousal. One of us worked with a carpenter who rigged an alarm to a winch that pulled him out of bed by the leg! Even if you do heed your alarm, you often experience such strong *sleep inertia*, with disorientation, leaden limbs, and persistent sleepiness, that it takes a long time to collect yourself and rise.

The last thing you feel like doing when you are finally on your feet is eat breakfast. The very thought of it may make you nauseous. When people with a delayed sleep phase are asked to log their food intake, it turns out that meals are delayed as well, with the first often taken after noon, and a second in the evening. What often stands in for a third meal is consumed quite late at night—a series of snacks that extends from, say, 10 P.M. to 2 A.M. If you try to shift your sleep earlier before this pattern of food consumption is addressed, you will miss out on some of this last "meal." Then you may toss and turn in bed due to hunger, in addition to your delayed sleep phase.

People with delayed sleep phase disorder are not ready to face the day, both literally and figuratively. They often experience *photophobia* during their first hours of wakefulness, reporting that daylight hurts their eyes and leads to headaches. Do you pull down the shades and hunker down indoors when the sun is bright? Do you wear dark glasses when you finally venture outdoors? These responses work directly against efforts to shift your sleep earlier. That is because daylight obtained in the first hours of wakefulness is the main way we advance our circadian clocks, whether they are running extra-slow or not. By waiting for several hours before getting any daylight, and then reducing what you do receive with sunglasses, you are removing the "backstop" that prevents your sleep from drifting later.

In chapter 4 we emphasized the interdependence of the sleep/wake cycle and mood. We pointed, for example, to the *diurnal mood variation* often seen in depression, wherein mood is particularly bleak in the morning hours while improving toward evening. There is a known association between depression and circadian phase delay. Yet even those of you who are not clinically depressed may still brighten up considerably in the evening.

We often hear patients say that the nighttime hours are "when I finally feel myself." High school students who are supposed to be catching a 6:30 A.M. bus get around to their homework near midnight, "because I'm finally able to concentrate." This certainly can look like procrastination to parents, and again, there may be a component of dithering. Nonetheless, the problems attending delayed circadian rhythms are generally more complicated than that simple explanation would have it.

SOCIAL RHYTHMS ARE SHIFTED, TOO

Changes in sleepiness, appetite, light tolerance, and mood act within you as an individual. But just as we could not survive a physical vacuum, we do not live in a social one. Our interactions with family and friends have their own rhythms, and it is in fact these two-way patterns that can offer up the most stubborn resistance when prodded to change. How we get along with people depends in large part on how we are feeling at the time. If internal rhythms bestow upon you more alertness and vitality at night, that's when you'll socialize. A sunny face may be the last thing you want to see in the morning.

Pen pals notwithstanding, friendship used to depend primarily on physical proximity. Now that video chatting, texting, and other new ways to communicate have rendered that notion quaint, friends flock together temporally as well as spatially. Those we hang out with not only share our interests, they also share our preferred hours of wakefulness. Of course, we don't get to choose our parents and siblings so as to ensure a good match in these respects. With close relatives, the best we can do is to learn patterns of approach and avoidance that yield a pleasant exchange, or at least keep the peace.

This social equilibrium is upset when you phase shift your sleep/wake cycle. After all, your friends are not about to shift theirs to match! They may well feel abandoned when their late-night messages go unanswered. At home, you may come to regret losing the quiet hours that staying up late afforded you. True, your late sleep schedule has exacted a big price at work or at school. Yet as important as paychecks and grades are, we social animals are especially wary of threatening our bonds of affiliation. These reservations must be addressed if you wish to successfully reset your clock.

We've learned from the foregoing that the timing of your sleep, whether early or late, is reinforced by your innate circadian physiology, acquired beliefs and behaviors, daily routines, and social interactions. Still, your sleep pattern is not set in stone. Let's take a look now at how it may be changed, even against these odds.

CHRONOTHERAPY: THE FIRST TREATMENT FOR DELAYED SLEEP/ WAKE PHASE DISORDER

Arthur Spielman was a coauthor of the original 1981 paper that described delayed sleep phase syndrome, and presented *chronotherapy*, a novel nonpharmacological treatment, to address it. Recognizing that it is much easier to get people who have trouble falling asleep in the first place to go to sleep *later* rather than earlier, chronotherapy asked them to live for about a week on an extra-long "day," of twenty-seven hours' duration. This was accomplished by scheduling bedtime progressively three hours later each night. For example, a teenager who habitually went to bed around 3 A.M. and rose at 11 A.M., thereby missing several periods of school every day, would, with the consent of her principal, first be stabilized on that very late pattern. As chronotherapy began, she would be assigned time in bed between 6 A.M. and 2 P.M. (three hours later on both ends than the baseline pattern) for her first "night." The next cycle, sleep would be scheduled between 9 A.M. to 5 P.M., then noon to 8 P.M., and so on around the clock, until it was positioned at the desired late evening to early morning hours.

While initial reports utilizing this procedure were very promising, over the years some problems have become apparent with chronotherapy. First off, there is a chance it will trigger a mood swing in people with underlying bipolar disorder. (The same caveat holds for timed exposure to bright light, the other major means of effecting phase shifts, discussed below.) However, a more general concern is that people undergoing chronotherapy on an outpatient basis often find it difficult to complete the treatment. They can generally negotiate the first several shifts with no problem, as staying up all night and even into the morning is second nature! But during the second half of the protocol, when asked to sleep in the afternoon and early evening hours, they may bail out.

This is likely due to both social and biological factors: at the midway point of chronotherapy, patients are being asked to sleep at the very time in which, for years, they were just starting to feel awake! There is a sense of being off-tempo, of missing out on the evening's activities as one's entire social circle is finally stirring. Plus, the biological clock is a *strong oscillator*; it displays inertia, resisting changes in the service of keeping us on track. So it cannot be relied upon to promote sleep that is now, say, twelve hours out of phase, after just four days of tinkering.

Finally, some chronotherapy patients who do manage to complete the protocol have a hard time "applying the brakes," stabilizing sleep in an earlier slot. Some slide right by the target and quickly reestablish their preferred late pattern. Others can maintain earlier bedtime hours for a while, but eventually drift later.

For all the above reasons, today we employ chronotherapy judiciously. We consider it when patients cannot fall asleep until morning—that is, when their sleep phase is already shifted halfway around the clock. Then we follow up with carefully timed exposure to bright light or melatonin—the new treatments of choice, to be discussed below—as well as behavioral interventions to stabilize the early pattern.

WHAT ABOUT JET THERAPY?

Michael, a fourteen-year-old, arrives with his distraught mother clutching his failing report card. He sits glumly as she explains how Michael has been reprimanded many times at school for tardiness, unexcused absences, inattention, and falling asleep in class. On school nights Michael usually goes to sleep around 3 A.M. He has to be virtually pulled out of bed at 7 A.M., just minutes before his bus arrives. On weekends he goes to bed even later, and rises spontaneously around noon.

After reviewing his sleep logs, we note that Michael is essentially living on Honolulu time, five hours behind Eastern Standard Time. Furthermore, his constant shifting between early weekday and late weekend rising times is leading to a sort of perpetual "jet lag." At this point Michael's face finally brightens. "Well, what if I just move to Hawaii?" he asks. "Will that solve the problem?"

Unfortunately, we have to dash the student's dream of a quick and pleasant fix. For a week or so Michael would indeed find himself able to fall asleep around the same time as his new Hawaiian neighbors, and able to rise with them in the morning. But eventually Michael's sleep would likely drift back to his old pattern, and he would end up making the same mad rush to a bus stop, albeit under a palm tree.

Despite Michael's disappointment, this news does contain a glimmer of hope for him, and for all of you who contend with circadian rhythm disorders. For, from the perspective of Michael's biological clock, once he has reestablished his late pattern in Hawaii, *he has phase-shifted five hours*. True, it's in the wrong direction (even later than before), but he could just as well have resettled in London and advanced his sleep phase five hours *earlier*. Stable phase shifts are evidently possible; we just have to learn what factors yield them in new time zones, and what might be done to mimic those same factors at home.

WHAT ELSE CHANGES WHEN WE CHANGE PLACES?

Clearly something special happens in faraway places! Let's take a look at all the things that change when we move to a new time zone, to get a sense of what it takes to produce a more lasting shift in circadian rhythms, and to understand why it is difficult but not impossible to accomplish such a shift at home.

First and foremost, at any one moment the level of daylight varies around the globe. The reason we even need time zones, of course, is that our planet's twenty-four-hour rotation sweeps sunlight from east to west, resulting in fluctuating levels of illumination at a given location. As the brightness of noon reigns in New York, dawn is breaking in Honolulu. So from the moment Michael landed there, his circadian clock would be exposed to the midday sun, the setting sun, the darkness of midnight, and the rising sun all about five hours later than his internal clock had been used to. We shall soon see how the timing of light exposure has a direct effect on the timing of our sleep phase. This is how the Hawaiian sun (working in concert with other factors) herds thousands of newly arrived vacationers onto Hawaiian time each week.

We learned earlier that the dimming light of sunset triggers the pineal gland in our brain to release melatonin. The later sunsets of Hawaii delay the onset of melatonin secretion, pushing new arrivals from the East Coast toward later sleep. Similarly, their levels of melatonin begin to peak later, keeping them asleep when folks back home are already beginning to wake up.

Finally, it may seem trivial that stores open and close, meals are served, sporting events kick off, and other entertainments are scheduled in a westward sweep across the Earth, aligned with the arc of the sun. That is, you can more or less plan your days and nights in a new location assuming the same hours of operation, expressed in local time, as back home. However, if you stay put, these social opportunities *do not automatically shift* just because you've made a decision to advance or delay your sleep phase. This, together with the fact that sunrise and sunset times do not suddenly shift to help your cause, go a long way toward explaining why resetting your internal clock remains a challenge at home, even though the science has been well worked out. Your favorite hangouts will continue to hum along late into the night without you, right up until closing time.

As noted, Michael was essentially already on Hawaiian time without having left New York. If his laggard SCN and late-night habits could have just been left at home, moving to Honolulu might have indeed solved Michael's problem. Unfortunately, however, both Michael's SCN and his habits would have been "carry-ons." So while the Hawaiian sun could be counted on to bring most newcomers around to Hawaiian time within a week, a pattern that would then be reinforced by island life, it would be a different story for Michael. His personal habits and social interactions, working in concert with his slow circadian clock, would eventually return him to a full-fledged night owl pattern in the islands.

You can probably see where we're going with this. While manipulations involving light exposure and melatonin form the core of any intervention aiming to phase-shift sleep, treatment will be a slog if you merely try to sleep at a new time in your old life. You will have to make all kinds of concrete changes in the ways in which you eat, work, socialize, exercise, and more. Perhaps most important, you will need to form a whole new notion *of when it is getting late.*

START WHERE YOU ARE, AND SHIFT SLOWLY

So, let's begin. First, choose starting times that will yield the best chance of getting some sleep. If you find it easier to sleep late, go ahead and choose a late bedtime. If you are currently nodding off after dinner and waking in the middle of the night, start with an early schedule. Don't try to get ahead of yourself and choose times that are already halfway toward your goal just because last Thursday you were able to fall and stay asleep during those particular hours.

This recommendation to *start off where you can sleep* is critical to success. You already know what happens when you try to follow advice to "just go to bed at a normal time." However, it also means that you should not embark on our program if you are facing suspension from school, or dismissal from work, with one more late arrival. You will need at least a few weeks to consolidate your new sleep pattern. If you've run out of time you may need to formally negotiate a period of forbearance until the next vacation break.

Even if you are not facing an ultimatum, you will still have to consult your calendar for upcoming weeks. Make sure there are no wedding receptions, doctor's appointments, concerts, or other events that would require you to drastically depart from your target bedtimes. After years of dealing with scheduling conflicts, it has probably become second nature for you to sleep as best you can around appointments. However, this is exactly one of the behaviors we are hoping to change. Now would be a good time to start giving priority to your sleep.

Second, cut your average time in bed a bit short, perhaps by thirty or sixty minutes. This will increase your homeostatic sleep drive, and keep your sleep more consolidated as it begins to shift. Cut bedtime from the part of the night when you already experience trouble sleeping (the beginning of the night for those of you with a delayed sleep phase, the end for you who have one that is advanced). That way, you'll minimize actual sleep loss while improving sleep efficiency. Over the course of treatment, you'll gradually slide this slightly compressed window for sleep in the desired direction, toward earlier or later hours.

Third, go slowly in shifting your sleep phase. True, in the laboratory shifts can be accomplished readily, especially under protocols in which subjects have no idea what time it is. And as we just discussed, the altered timing of light exposure and social cues that occurs in a new time zone can produce relatively rapid shifts. That is why it only takes about one day to adapt to each hour of time zone change following jet travel.

However, in your own home town, where nothing has changed but your determination to live on a new schedule, you should aim to shift in half-hour, or even quarter-hour, increments. Furthermore, hold to interim times for at least several nights before making another shift. After all, your goal is not merely to demonstrate that you can sleep at a particular time and move on. Many of you do that all the time. It is about *stabilizing* sleep on an earlier or later pattern. You would do better to experience some stability, even if on a modestly altered schedule, right away.

USE BRIGHT LIGHT TO **PUSH** SLEEP AWAY

As we have seen, appropriately timed light exposure, the core ingredient for successful phase shifting, is supplied automatically when you move to a new time zone. At home you'll have to provide for yourself. Exposure to bright light can either delay or advance the timing of your sleep, depending upon when that exposure occurs in relation to your usual sleep time. A handy way to think about it is that light *repels* sleep. If you are exposed to bright light before retiring in the evening, it will tend to push your sleep phase later, further away from the time you were getting the light. If, on the other hand, you are exposed to bright light soon after awakening in the morning, it will tend to push your sleep phase earlier, again away from the time when light is obtained.

Before we get into the specifics of treatment, a few words of precaution are in order. Bright light, whether from the sun or a light box (a device that produces intense light to mimic the circadian effects of sunlight), can pose special risks for people with a number of medical conditions, as well as for those who are taking certain medications. These include:

- Conditions that render the eyes more vulnerable to damage from bright light, including macular degeneration and retinal dystrophies.
- Medical disorders that increase sensitivity to light, such as porphyria and lupus, or a history of skin cancer.
- Medications that increase sensitivity to light, including the phenothiazines, antiarrhythmic drugs such as Amiodarone, and St. John's wort.
- A history of bipolar disorder, given clinical evidence that bright light treatment can trigger manic or hypomanic episodes.

This list is not meant to be comprehensive; it merely serves to underscore the point that everyone who is considering light therapy, whether via a light box or natural light, should first consult with their healthcare provider to determine whether the treatment can be safely administered.

You very late sleepers have a choice when it comes to obtaining appropriately timed bright light. The sun is at least up when you need it—soon after awakening—even if it's perhaps the last thing you want to see! Cloudy days, by the way, do not provide you an excuse to skip treatment. There is still generally enough light for our purposes. If, however, you are reading these words on a frigid day in January, you would do well to purchase a light box to allow for consistent indoor bright light exposure. Whether under a light box or under the sun, you'll want to set aside about thirty minutes for light treatment.

If you have an advanced sleep phase, finding yourself very sleepy in the evening and prone to early morning awakenings, you would benefit from evening light exposure. There has been less systematic work on the effects of evening light therapy, and studies often involved prolonged exposure times that would be impractical in a home setting. Yet there are theoretical reasons to suspect that longer exposures may be necessary then: since treatment takes place many hours before the core body temperature reaches its minimum, it has a less potent phase-shifting effect. You can take a long evening stroll if it happens to be summertime. Otherwise you will definitely need a light box. Plan to obtain about one hour's light exposure nightly, starting in the midevening and ending at least one hour before you turn in.

Light boxes are available from numerous vendors in the $100 to $300 range. At recommended working distances, current light boxes typically provide intensities of 5,000 or 10,000 lux (a unit of measurement of light intensity on a surface), compared to typical indoor illuminations of just a few hundred lux. Preferred units are mounted on stands to illuminate from an angle slightly above your line of vision. If your light box rests directly on the table, make sure to position it away from your direct line of sight, slightly off to the left or the right, typically at about arm's length. It will not work if it is aimed at the side of your face, stationed in the corner of the room while you are moving about, or, need we say, shining down while you continue to sleep with your head buried under a pillow!

Early research with light boxes used white light. About fifteen years ago it was discovered that our circadian system is maximally responsive to blue light, so some units are now tuned specifically to emit light in the blue range. It is not clear that these provide any additional benefit, since white light is composed of wavelengths from across the visual spectrum, including the blue portion. Regardless of what color light is emitted, be sure to obtain a light device with adequate filtering of harmful ultraviolet light. Understand that even units employing optimal filters and diffusers will still allow a very small amount of ultraviolet light to come through, so please carefully follow the manufacturer's recommendations. In any case, you should never stare at a source of very bright light, whether it is the sun or a light box. You do, however, need to keep your eyes open as you look elsewhere!

REMOVE BRIGHT LIGHT (OR AT LEAST BLUE LIGHT) WHEN IT'S WORKING AGAINST YOU

The discovery that the circadian clock is selectively responsive to light in the blue portion of the visual spectrum has led to new phase-shifting strategies. Goggles or wraparound sunglasses with amber lenses block blue light, and thereby fool the internal clock into thinking it is in the dark, even though there is still plenty of light available for vision. You can position blue-blocking glasses on the opposite side of your sleep, compared to when you are obtaining light exposure, to facilitate a phase shift.

For example, if you are obtaining morning light to advance your delayed sleep phase, you could also wear blue-blocking glasses in the evening, especially when outdoors on long summer days. You could use them when staring at your computer screen in the evening any time of year. However, there is a more elegant solution available to block screen light—programs such as f.lux that disable the blue pixels after sunset. These programs rely on the computer's clock and stored information on seasonal daylight patterns to appropriately time the change of screen color.

If you are already awakening too early, bright light exposure in the morning will worsen the problem. So those of you with an advanced sleep phase would likely benefit from wearing blue-blocking glasses if you go outdoors after sunrise. While this application is more commonly recommended for the elderly, we have also suggested blue-blocking glasses for younger athletes who aim to awaken at, say, 6:30 A.M. for a morning run but who find themselves awakening at 5:30 A.M. or even 4:30 A.M. instead. These runners are inadvertently triggering a phase advance with their consistent early light exposure.

USE MELATONIN TO **PULL** SLEEP CLOSER

We have discussed how the pineal gland in the brain begins to secrete the hormone melatonin as the sky dims. If artificial light does not inhibit this natural reaction to increasing darkness, the level of internally produced, or *endogenous*, melatonin rises rapidly. About four hours later, as it nears its peak, we generally feel ready to turn in. Melatonin plateaus at a relatively high concentration during the first couple of hours of our sleep. It then begins a steady decline, so that only a small amount of endogenous melatonin remains by the time we typically awaken.

Before we discuss how you might use melatonin to shift your sleep, we should emphasize that although oral melatonin is available at every vitamin and health food store, and may therefore be perceived as totally benign, it is a hormone with complex activity in the body. It has not been as rigorously studied as medications that must obtain FDA approval. Even though decades of clinical use, and more recent systematic research, indicate that it can be used safely and effectively, it may also lead to daytime hangover, dizziness, mood disturbance, gastrointestinal complaints, and other problems. Melatonin may interfere with the functioning of birth control pills, blood thinners, and other medications. For all these reasons, you should discuss any potential use of melatonin with your healthcare provider beforehand, and together assess both its effectiveness and its side effects.

The sleep phase-shifting effect of exogenous melatonin is the opposite of that produced by light. Evening melatonin *pulls* the sleep phase earlier, toward the time of ingestion, so it can be useful for those of you prone to sleeping very late. Morning melatonin *pulls* the sleep phase later, again toward the time of ingestion, so it would be the choice for you who find yourselves sleeping too early.

The phase-shifting effect of melatonin can be accomplished with small doses of 0.3 mg or 0.5 mg, as well as with the 3 mg dose that is commonly employed when melatonin is taken as a sleep aid at bedtime. This is likely so because when melatonin is administered to shift a sleep phase, either in the early evening or the morning, the brain contains minimal endogenous levels of the substance. The "dusk signal," the first secretion of melatonin that the pineal gland naturally secretes in response to dimming light, is itself vanishingly small.

We recommend that you first try facilitating your shift with a 0.3 mg or 0.5 mg dose. That way you are more likely to avoid feeling sleepy during waking hours. It can be difficult to find such small melatonin dosages locally, although some national vitamin store chains do sell a 1 mg pill that can be cut in pieces. They are also available on the internet; several formulations may be found, for example, on Amazon. Note that 0.3 mg may be labeled as 300 mcg (300 micrograms). Make sure to buy a synthetic or "vegetarian" formulation.

What time you should take melatonin so as to yield the largest phase shift is a bit complicated to work out at home. It depends on your endogenous melatonin rhythm, the average length of your sleep, and the dosage of melatonin you take. Fortunately, Helen Burgess and colleagues have come up with some good rules of thumb that you can employ by keeping a sleep log for a week or two and then calculating the average midpoint of your sleep. Using the 0.5 dosage, the optimal time to administer melatonin to help pull your sleep forward is a little more than ten hours *before* this midpoint, which for most people will be about five or six hours before bedtime. For example, if you have a delayed sleep phase and normally sleep from about 4 A.M.

to noon, the midpoint of your sleep will be around 8 A.M. You should therefore take 0.5 mg melatonin at 10 P.M., that is, six hours before your bedtime.

Morning melatonin at 0.5 mg taken about six-and-a-half hours *after* the sleep midpoint most effectively pulls the sleep phase later. So if you are now sleeping, on average, from 8 P.M. to 3 A.M., the midpoint of your current sleep phase is 11:30 P.M., and you may want to take melatonin around 6 A.M.

Note that in some cases of early morning awakening, especially in the elderly, it may be that the pineal gland is simply not secreting enough melatonin. Clinicians have therefore experimented with having patients take melatonin at the time of awakening, with the aim of extending sleep. This is not specifically a circadian rhythm issue, but we touch on it here to avoid confusion if you come across these instructions elsewhere. Timed release melatonin, taken at bedtime, is also used in such circumstances.

WAKING LIFE PUSHES AND PULLS AT SLEEP TOO

Bright light and melatonin may be the main levers that prod our sleep earlier or later, but they are by no means the only ones. We have seen that virtually every facet of daily living can push or pull at sleep. If the timing of meals, especially, does not change, it will resist your efforts to sleep at a new hour. This can be harder to accomplish than swallowing melatonin or switching on a light box. You will need to make a concerted effort to gradually shift caloric intake.

The first step, for those with a delayed sleep phase, is just to admit to the possibility that you, of all people, can eat breakfast. The next is to begin a ritual of sitting down at the kitchen table soon after awakening for a minimeal—even if initially it consists of a few cereal flakes or half a slice of toast with coffee or juice. Similarly, you can no longer consider a power bar obtained from a vending machine to be lunch; you'll need to do better than that. As more of your caloric intake starts to migrate earlier in the day, you'll want to cut back on how much you consume after dinner. A light snack is okay close to your still-delayed bedtime. However, you will have to forsake that pattern of constant nocturnal grazing in front of a TV or computer screen if you want to eventually be sleeping rather than eating at night.

Just as there is inertia when it comes to budging our appetites, it takes some diplomacy to revamp our social calendars without ruffling feathers or worse, losing friends. Fortunately, face time need not all be lost. You can still go out late with your friends on weekends, even if you may have to beg off at some point rather than hitting the after-party. Of course, rather than sleeping in all morning, you will want to limit yourself to one extra hour, and then get some light! You should, however, change their expectations that you'll take their calls, answer their texts, and respond to their posts at all hours. If you can explain your motivations ahead of time and head off any perceived snubs, maybe your friends will return the favor—they just might let you get some sleep at night.

CHAPTER SUMMARY

- Our preferred timing for sleeping has a biological basis—an internal circadian clock, the suprachiasmatic nucleus. The timing of this clock typically runs a bit slow relative to the Earth's twenty-four-hour rotation, but it varies among individuals by more than an hour.

- Mistimed circadian clocks compel us to reset our internal rhythms every cycle in order to stay on a schedule, much as one would adjust the hands on an antique clock that ran slow or fast. Individuals with fast internal clocks tend toward early sleep schedules. Those with extra-slow clocks, the more commonly seen variant, have delayed sleep, living as "night owls."

- A delayed sleep phase often results in reprimands at school or work for tardiness. This in turn can spur overlays of frustration, helplessness, and reduced motivation. Yet at its core the problem remains based on an inherited trait, which should prompt some accommodation.

- The circadian clock does not directly put us to sleep. Rather, it opens a window for the best opportunity to sleep—by timing core body temperature, hormone release, and many other physiological rhythms. It is linked to the light/dark cycle by the release of melatonin at dusk.

- In addition to regulating sleep, the circadian clock profoundly influences your waking day. It affects when you will be most active, most likely exposed to outdoor light, and at your best in terms of mood, productivity, and sociability. Although these waking preferences become ingrained, they must also be shifted, if you wish to successfully retime your sleep.

- The most successful sleep phase shifts occur after moving to a new time zone. New hours of daylight, relative to what your internal clock expected, powerfully entrain the new schedule. Social cues all change their timing in unison, reinforcing the shift. None of these factors budge, however, when you try to shift your sleep at home. That's why it is hard to do.

- Begin your phase shift where you are best able to sleep. Gradually move time in bed earlier or later by fifteen or thirty minutes, holding to interim schedules for a few days. Use bright light to push sleep, while blocking blue light and taking melatonin to pull sleep, in the desired direction. Plan your meals, activities, appointments, and socializing to reinforce the new pattern.

- Those of you wishing to phase delay sleep will be challenged not only to remain awake but also to imagine yourself engaged in evening activities. Those wishing to phase advance must work against a powerful sense that staying up very late "is natural," and come to think of morning as a time to get things done. While circadian science can certainly help shift your sleep phase, the shift that takes place in your mind may well be what proves decisive.

CHAPTER SEVEN

Are You Too **Dependent on Medication** for Sleep?

While chronic insomnia triggers all kinds of distress, perhaps none is as acute as the anxiety faced by those of you who believe that medication is necessary for sleep. Your apprehension may center on securing a continuous supply of sleeping pills in the face of reluctant physicians and ever-stricter insurance limitations. You may feel especially aggravated because you can sleep well enough, so long as you take your medicine. Other people are routinely prescribed their statins and their antihypertensives. Why, you ask, do you have to jump through hoops to treat your sleep disorder?

Others of you may be more ambivalent about relying on hypnotics. Perhaps you have read about, or experienced firsthand, the memory impairments, nocturnal falls, morning hangovers, or other problems associated with such medication. As their drawbacks emerge, you are beginning to question your habit of taking sleep aids practically every night. You may have heard about epidemiological studies linking increased mortality with the use of sleeping pills, and are all the more confused by conflicting expert opinions rendered on this dire claim. Now you find yourself facing the unenviable choice of either medicated sleep associated with all sorts of risks, or else making do with insomnia, which of course brings its own special miseries and, yes, health hazards.

The majority of our readers are likely to be caught up in still another sleep aid dilemma. You've made your peace with the potential side effects of these medications, but unlike the first group described, you are not particularly enamored of them. That is because the sleep you get with pills is mediocre at best. You'd be glad to give them up for good, but whenever you try, you hardly sleep at all! After several hours of tossing and turning, you give in and take a dose, to salvage what remains of the night. By now you've been through this drill so often that just the thought of trying to sleep on your own is enough to get your heart racing. How can you be expected to sleep when you're forever on the verge of a panic attack?

We know we are working under a certain selection bias here. There are many people who do well over the long term on sleeping pills, perhaps taking them intermittently throughout the month, or even nightly during particularly stressful stretches. Their treatment takes place under the watchful eyes of doctors and nurses, who are comfortable maintaining such prudent usage. It's just that as insomnia treatment specialists working in sleep disorder centers, we don't see many of these satisfied drug responders walking through our door—and as authors, we do not anticipate them opening our book. So it is to all of you who have weighed the personal pros and cons of sleeping pills with your providers, and who are now looking to reduce your dependency on medication, that we here offer encouragement and advice.

As psychologists practicing in New York State, we do not ourselves prescribe medication. For decades, though, we have been working with medical colleagues to help our mutual patients optimize their use of hypnotics when indicated, and minimize that usage when not. This collaboration typically includes discussing the effects of various medication choices on sleep, monitoring their side effects, and facilitating tapering protocols. Oftentimes we will institute behavioral interventions to strengthen both the sleep and the confidence of our hypnotic-reliant patients, before any gradual withdrawal is begun. To set the stage for *your* taper we first wish to discuss, from the perspective of behavioral sleep specialists, just how your sleeping pills succeed when they work well, and why they fail when they don't.

DOES SLEEP COME FROM YOU OR THE PILL?

Psychologists use the term "locus of control" to describe the extent to which people believe they can influence the events occurring in their lives. Usually this concept is fairly straightforward: people with an external locus believe that things happen due to forces beyond their control. According to this way of thinking, what happens was bound to happen, and there isn't much anyone can do about it. By contrast, those with an internal locus of control believe that their efforts and actions exert at least some influence on the course of events.

Our perceived locus of control influences how actively we pursue our objectives. The issue often boils down to: should we make the effort or not? In most of life's endeavors, more concerted effort is more likely to be rewarded with success. This usually confers an advantage on those with an internal locus of control. At first glance, sleep would seem to present an exception to this rule, since it doesn't typically respond to direct effort.

For example, Jasmin prides herself on taking action to solve problems, both at home and on the job. When she began to experience trouble falling asleep, Jasmin assigned herself a strict bedtime of 9:30 P.M. and made a point of getting home right after work, so as to secure a four-hour wind-down period prior to getting into bed. During the evening she tried to avoid, as much as possible, physical exertion, social stimulation, and intellectual engagement. She opted for an expensive high-tech mattress, even though her current one was not very old and seemed serviceable. Each night she made sure the sheets covering her new bed were fresh, spread a lavender scent, and cooled the room to sixty-eight degrees. To complete her blitz of preparation, Jasmin donned an eye mask and started up a device producing sounds of steady rainfall. Yet despite Jasmin's best efforts to bring sleep under her control, it refused to fall into line.

What's going on here? No doubt some of Jasmin's interventions were helpful. The sleep environment *should* be comfortable, and fashioning a bedtime ritual *can* soothe adults to sleep, just as it does for children. It should be said, however, that some of Jasmin's choices were more questionable, such as her prolonged buffer period. Remaining sedentary and unstimulated for four hours each evening blunts the circadian peak of alertness, and can lead to a "second wind" when bedtime finally comes around.

However, the bigger problem is that Jasmin's locus of control really isn't internal. It is quite likely that *she still believes herself to be a poor sleeper*, who in fact needs all kinds of special arrangements before she can nod off. An internal locus is better represented by someone who is just quietly confident that she sleeps well under most conditions. When poor sleep does occur, she doesn't give it too much thought, but might note that anyone can have a bad night.

Relying on sleeping pills is perhaps the most extreme example of relocating control of sleep to an external source. This may be because there is nothing about pills that corresponds to any natural human preference for sleep. Blankets feel warm and soft next to the skin—they are truly "sleep aids." Pillows support the neck; even eyeshades and white noise generators work to relieve our senses of their propensity to respond to environmental stimuli. By contrast, the perceived physical attributes of pills are designed not for sleeping, but for swallowing. They seem to be little seeds of sleep itself, which need only be ingested to work their wonders within us, no collaboration necessary.

This is a major misconception that can lead to serious consequences. As with Jasmin, our zealous insomniac, those of you who are hypnotic dependent also regard yourselves as "poor sleepers," with the difference that you are intent not on securing a perfect sleep environment but a prescription. Whereas Jasmin could at least turn over her pillow, adjust her eyeshades, or engage in a host of other maneuvers when she found herself unable to sleep, your only recourse may be to either tough it out or reach for a pill. Let's consider all that happens when you choose the latter course of action.

PHARMACOLOGICAL ACTIVITY OF SLEEPING PILLS

Hypnotic medications are active substances, products of an increasingly sophisticated understanding of how alterations in brain chemistry affect sleep. Most hypnotic drugs developed to date have worked within pathways utilizing the neurotransmitter gamma aminobutyric acid, or GABA, which generally has an inhibiting effect in the brain.

In the course of this development, the benzodiazepine hypnotics such as triazolam (Halcion), temazepam (Restoril), and flurazepam (Dalmane) represented a major advance over the earlier barbiturates such as secobarbital (Seconal) in terms of safety. Similarly, newer hypnotics such as zolpidem (Ambien) and eszopiclone (Lunesta), which are not benzodiazepines but which bind to the same receptors, are able to induce sleep with fewer unwanted consequences such as the "morning hangover" that was especially problematic with some of the longer-acting benzodiazepine drugs. Most recently, sleep aids have been developed that exploit other sleep-regulatory mechanisms, including the melatonin receptor agonist ramelteon (Rozerem) and the orexin receptor antagonist suvorexant (Belsomra).

Concerns raised by the most widely prescribed hypnotics have not been so much over their safety or effectiveness but rather over their effects on functions other than sleep—that is, their side effect profile. A major goal of hypnotic drug development has been to formulate medications that promote sleep but not much else. Given that sleep as a brain function involves some of the same chemical messengers that regulate mood, appetite, cognition, muscle tone, arousal, and other essential functions, attaining such specificity of action has been an ongoing challenge.

PSYCHOLOGICAL ACTIVITY OF SLEEPING PILLS

As pharmaceutical companies home in on the trifecta of safety, efficacy, and specificity, they have not paid as much attention to the unique psychological context in which hypnotic drugs are consumed. In controlled clinical trials, the demonstrated ability of the current crop of hypnotics to get people asleep and keep them sleeping is fairly modest: their advantages over placebo in these core metrics are typically measured in fractions of an hour. These results may speak more to the particular power of placebos when it comes to matters of sleep than they discount the effectiveness of medication.

We think that placebos make surprisingly good showings in hypnotic drug trials in part because *the act of taking a pill*, whether medication or placebo, tends to free poor sleepers of their efforts to sleep. Placebo effects are of course ubiquitous throughout medicine. However, as we have emphasized throughout this book, fervently trying to fall asleep tends to be an especially counterproductive strategy. Once a pill is ingested, a psychic handoff takes place: responsibility for sleep is transferred to the pill, and even if that pill is composed of sugar this act of standing down is nearly as important as lying down, insofar as inducing sleep is concerned.

You probably have personal experience that corroborates this claim. Think back to all those occasions when, after tottering on the brink of sleep for hours, you finally took a sleeping pill, and promptly fell asleep. While modern hypnotics are formulated for a rapid onset of action, and a quick buildup to peak levels, they are not *that* fast. They are not putting you to sleep within two or three minutes.

The reason you fell asleep so quickly is more likely that the homeostatic and circadian sleep regulatory mechanisms working in your favor when you took a pill at, say, 1:30 A.M. were finally able to engage. By then, you might have been awake for eighteen or nineteen hours, and had built up a strong drive for sleep. Your core body temperature would have been rapidly falling towards its nadir, a circadian phase that produces little alerting force to oppose the increased homeostatic drive.

In fact, with so much drive for sleep, and so little alerting force to resist it, you might ask why you didn't just fall asleep before you could even reach for the pill. At that juncture, your wakefulness was being enforced by *hyperarousal*, the main theme of chapter 2, acting as an "emergency override." Finding yourself once more unable to sleep had in essence morphed into a crisis. Just as hyperarousal would awaken you in a hurry if your bedroom window shattered in the middle of the night, no matter how fast asleep you were, prior to swallowing the pill hyperarousal was masking your underlying sleepiness. Your desperation for sleep was, in effect, keeping you from tipping over its edge.

When this hyperarousal was assuaged by the act of taking a pill, it was as if floodgates were lifted. You exchanged agitation and despair that you would ever get to sleep for hope that *the pill would bring sleep to you*, and ceased your worrying and your efforts. Sure enough, once you finally allowed yourself to relax, the latent sleepiness that had been building all along proved overwhelming.

GIVE YOURSELF SOME CREDIT

This scenario, played out repeatedly, explains why many of you are convinced you need hypnotic medication. Too often sleep seems to make its appearance at random: one night you fall off just fine despite having had coffee after dinner, but the next, after spending a strenuous day outdoors, you lie awake for hours. So when something as seemingly clear-cut as falling asleep minutes after ingesting a sleeping pill occurs, you are only too eager to assign cause and effect. Still, who did the heavy lifting here? True, the pill may have augmented your propensity for sleep, but it was riding the crest of a homeostatic drive that *you yourself* had created by being awake all day and half the night. It was also taking advantage of favorable circadian circumstances, coasting down from the peak of a rhythm that *you yourself* built up over preceding weeks and months.

If you doubt the magnitude of your contribution, think about how much extra sleep that same sleeping pill generates when you are not helping it out. For example, many of you may recall a particularly horrendous night when, totally exasperated and frantic, you popped a sleeping pill near morning. Do you sleep anywhere near eight hours from that point? No, in such circumstances you would be lucky to get just a few hours, usually followed by a serious case of drug hangover.

More reasonably, when eastward air travel lands you in a new time zone after nightfall, you may decide to take a sleeping pill before turning in. After all, it may still be just late afternoon at home. You could hardly be expected to get a full quotient of sleep at that time of day. With your drug you can induce a few hours of sleep to appear earlier than they would otherwise. However, the middle of the night may be punctuated with arousals, since your internal clock still thinks it is evening, and you are generally pretty alert during evening hours. Eventually your circadian rhythms are ready to help you sleep again, because it is finally night back home. Of course, by then day is breaking in your new locale, and it can be particularly difficult to rouse yourself.

WHEN SLEEPING PILLS LET YOU DOWN

We have seen that the relaxation that comes of handing off responsibility for sleep to a pill, in combination with that pill's pharmacology, can lead to rapid slumber. Given this potent mixture, the question arises why sleeping pills don't work for you more consistently.

The more straightforward pitfalls are pharmacological. Chronic hypnotic administration usually leads to a decrease in drug effectiveness, whether after weeks, months, or years. The particular interval in which a drug remains effective depends upon the frequency and dosage of administration, the type of medication employed, and individual differences in drug sensitivity. There is also a pharmacological basis for the "rebound insomnia" that occurs upon abrupt withdrawal from sleeping pills (in addition to psychological factors stemming from the knowledge that one is not taking a full dose). Many drug effects are temporarily reversed upon withdrawal; in the case of sleeping pills sedating and hypnotic effects give way to increased anxiety and arousal.

The upshot of these expected pharmacological effects is that, when hypnotic medications are used nightly, strong initial improvements in sleep quantity and quality moderate somewhat, before a stable plateau is reached. This plateau is your "drugged sleep." Whether it is of good quality or just so-so, if you judge that sleep to be better than what you can expect without medication, you may become reliant on pills. (In practice, this judgment is often rendered between sleep with medications and the first few nights off of them, which, due to rebound insomnia, is not a fair comparison.)

It should be mentioned here that one popular benzodiazepine receptor agonist, Lunesta, was seen in a controlled study that used subjective measures of sleep quality to still be demonstrating improvement over placebo after six months. That said, in practice many patients feel that Lunesta, like other sleep aids, is most effective initially. We suspect that individual differences play a large role in how patients respond to all long-term hypnotic administration, but in general it should be expected that some degree of tolerance to sleeping pills will build over time.

Problems also occur when you do not collaborate with your medicine, when you believe yourself absolved of all responsibility for sleep. To do well with hypnotics, you still have to do a fair amount of work: You have to build up your sleep drive by refraining from daytime naps and from over-sleeping. You have to entrain a strong circadian sleep/wake cycle by positioning your sleep phase in approximately the same time slot each night, and especially by awakening at the same time each morning to receive consistently timed daylight exposure. You have to bring yourself down gradually from active engagement with the day, ending with an hour or so of a "buffer period" of quiet activity such as reading, without actually dipping into sleep. Relying on sleeping pills can make you lazy in all these regards.

In sum, reliance on sleeping pills may allow you to relax about sleep—which is a good thing tonight—but it also renders you more lax about sleep, which is not so helpful in the long run. In a paradox worthy of a Zen koan, out-sourcing responsibility for slumber to something outside yourself (in this case to a small pill), can end up reinforcing your sense of having insomnia while at the same time it brings sleep. In the next section we will discuss how to use medication while retaining accountability for your sleep, for those times when you and your provider have decided that drug treatment is the right choice. We follow with suggestions that can facilitate a successful taper off medication, when you are ready to sleep on your own.

WHEN DO SLEEP AIDS MAKE SENSE?

Even though we have both spent decades promoting behavioral treatments for insomnia, we believe that some situations call for at least considering a front-line use of sleep aids. Acute life disruptions, such as losing a loved one or surviving a natural disaster, are prime indications. Traumatic events trigger emergency hyperarousal responses and immediately make a claim on all our strength and coping skills. They are best met with as much sleep as we can muster from the get-go. And while the effects of such disruptions will certainly linger, the first weeks are often the hardest—a time span that jibes nicely with recommended guidelines for most hypnotic usage. Other periods of elevated stress hardly qualifying as catastrophic but which have definite endpoints, such as the weeks before a product launch, or even a wedding, may trigger sleeplessness that is reasonably addressed with medication.

What favors the use of sleeping pills in times of crisis or acute stress is that such periods are by definition readily distinguished from the norm. That is, while they are part of life, they are not part of what we think of as *daily life*. If we resort to the use of medication at such times, we are not taking pills simply because we are unable to sleep but rather because we are unable to sleep under such trying conditions. The distinction may seem a fine one, but it becomes very important when processes of acclimation eventually begin to soothe our loss, or the big event triggering our anticipatory anxiety finally arrives. We recognize that our days are easing, and this brings an expectation that our nights will, too. After all, in our time of stress we knew all too well what to blame for our poor sleep, and it was not ourselves.

There are many factors that weigh against the use of hypnotics, even in times of crisis. These medications present special risks for the elderly, who may metabolize the drugs more slowly, be prone to falls, or be showing mild cognitive impairment. Younger adults whose jobs or caretaking duties keep them on-call at night, who labor under hazardous conditions, who cosleep with young children, or who have demonstrated addiction to other substances, are likewise more at risk, given the dissociated states, morning sleepiness, and drug dependency that can occur as side effects of hypnotic usage.

WHAT KIND OF SLEEP AID SHOULD YOU USE?

If you and your provider have agreed that a medication trial is indicated, the next step might be a discussion of which type would be best for your given situation. We believe that there is still a strong case to be made for hypnotics, which, after all, were specifically developed to promote sleep. Their effectiveness has been demonstrated in placebo-controlled, randomized clinical trials. They do a good job of preserving normal sleep architecture while reducing nocturnal wakefulness and minimizing morning hangover effects.

Nonetheless, hypnotic medications are not the only or even the most widely employed choices. Despite a general lack of controlled clinical studies attesting to their effectiveness for treating insomnia, physicians have long prescribed medications that produce sleepiness as a side effect for their patients with sleep complaints. Common examples include the alpha-2 adrenergic agonist clonidine, relied upon by pediatricians for treatment of sleep problems in children, or the sedating antidepressants trazodone, amitriptyline, and doxepin, used by many general practitioners for adults.

Newer antidepressants that include a noradrenergic action among their effects, such as mirtazapine (Remeron), are also being used today to address insomnia, in contrast to such first-generation selective serotonin reuptake inhibitors (SSRIs) as fluoxetine (Prozac), which often led to increased sleep disruption. In still other cases, providers may aim to reduce anxiety levels in the hours before sleep, with anxiolytic medication such as the benzodiazepines alprazolam (Xanax) or clonazepam (Klonopin).

Over-the-counter medications have also proven very popular treatments for sleep. Antihistamines such as diphenhydramine (Benadryl, Tylenol PM) and doxylamine succinate (Unisom) block the histamine response that leads to allergic symptoms, but with concomitant sleepiness that has led to their widespread use as sleep aids. While there is a natural tendency to give the benefit of the doubt to venerable treatments that have been available without prescription from corner drugstores for generations, antihistamines are not without drawbacks. Most common are daytime drowsiness, a result of these drugs' relatively long half-life (that of diphenhydramine averages over eight hours, with substantially longer durations seen in the elderly), dizziness, and dry mouth.

Memory problems have long been seen as a potential issue with anticholinergic medications, including the antihistamines discussed above. In addition to clinical experience with these drugs yielding cognitive complaints, basic research has demonstrated a central role for the neurotransmitter acetylcholine in learning and memory. Long-term usage of drugs that strongly block cholinergic activity in the brain might therefore be expected to affect memory.

Even given these considerations, a study published by Shelly Gray and colleagues in *JAMA Internal Medicine* in 2015 demonstrating that cumulative use of anticholinergic medication over ten years was linked to increased risk for the development of dementia caused quite a stir both in clinical circles and in the popular press. This study was conducted in a group of over 3,400 primarily white college-educated subjects, aged sixty-five or older when their participation began. Cognitive functioning was assessed every two years, over an average follow-up period of over seven years. Subjects who frequently used anticholinergic medication in commonly prescribed doses were at greater risk for developing dementia, compared to those who did not often use such drugs, and a strong dose-response relationship was observed.

While these results of course await replication, and generalization in other populations, they underscore the need to consider risk-benefit ratios in all medications, whether prescription or over the counter. It should be added here that the antidepressants amitriptyline (Elavil) and doxepin (Sinequan) also have strong anticholinergic effects, whereas this is less of an issue with trazodone (Desyrel).

WHAT'S YOUR EXIT STRATEGY?

One of the reasons antihistamines, sedating antidepressants, and the sleep-inducing hormone melatonin are enlisted to address insomnia is that they are seen as "non-habit-forming," that is, less likely to lead to drug dependence. It is true that people generally do not crave these substances. They do not typically lead to a marked change in mood, whether euphoria or calm, and their side effects, especially with regard to morning hangover, would dissuade most people from increasing dosages beyond suggested limits.

However, while these are credible safeguards insofar as traditional views of drug dependence are concerned, they do not take into account the special psychological challenges posed by the use of sleep aids. As discussed, we tend to give the credit for sleep to the pills we take, of whatever type, which in turn renders us increasingly doubtful of our ability to sleep without them. So when sleep aids can be obtained over the counter, the resulting combination of easy accessibility and perceived harmlessness can make them seem perfect for everlasting use.

For those of you who are suffering from insomnia together with depression or anxiety, the use of sedating antidepressant or anxiolytic medications may well constitute an effective and efficient treatment approach. In these cases, pharmacological treatment is best coupled with CBT-I so as to address difficulties initiating or maintaining sleep that can persist beyond resolution of the mood or anxiety disorder. For the rest of you, who are contending primarily with insomnia, we see a reasonable strategy as one that may resort to some type of hypnotic medication in acute crises, and to cognitive behavioral treatments when precipitating factors have subsided but sleeplessness has not.

TAKING THE PILL: TIMING IS KEY

Taking a sleeping pill would seem sufficiently straightforward to avoid the need for further discussion, but in fact we see all kinds of departures from recommended practice. Perhaps the most common is waiting an hour or two to see if sleep will come "naturally" before finally giving up and swallowing the medicine. Although this pattern may stem from a laudable motivation to cut down on the number of pills consumed per week, in practice it doesn't yield so much a reduction in usage as a reduction in hours of sleep.

If you recognize this pattern as your own, you have essentially conditioned yourself to stay awake for a while before taking a sleeping pill. There really isn't much decision making involved. The decision you *should* be making with your doctor is whether pharmacotherapy is indicated, and if so, how often and for how long you should take your medicine. Once that is decided (and while helping your sleeping pill help you, through all the cognitive and behavioral means we've reviewed), the best course is to just follow your treatment plan, and take your pill at lights out or shortly before.

Of course, for those of you suffering primarily from difficulty maintaining sleep, your treatment plan may *specify* middle-of-the-night drug administration. The hypnotic Intermezzo, containing a smaller dose of zolpidem formulated to dissolve under the tongue, has been developed to treat such sleep-maintenance insomnia. Among other precautions, Intermezzo should be taken only when you have at least four hours of bedtime remaining, and can then be up and about for an additional hour before driving.

A second common drug-taking practice, which errs in the opposite direction, is trying to get "a running start" toward sleep by taking your pill more than an hour before retiring. This pattern is problematic in several ways. Foremost are the risks of falling or acting dangerously while in a dissociated state before you turn in. There have been many news stories over the years to remind us that even when people are supposedly safely in bed, the use of hypnotic medication increases the probability of parasomnia activity and injury. This risk is magnified when you have not yet retired, while a drug is already working to get you to sleep.

In addition to safety concerns, taking your sleeping pill too early reduces its effectiveness. Most hypnotic medications are fast-acting, attaining peak plasma levels within an hour to an hour and a half. When you take a pill two hours before getting into bed, you squander much of the drug's benefit before you are finally ready to sleep. And if the pill triggers microsleeps while you are waiting, you also squander some of the homeostatic sleep drive that would better serve you by consolidating sleep later that night. Finally, you set yourself up for an early morning awakening as the drug's hypnotic effect wanes. So if you are going to use a sleeping pill at all, our recommendation would be to allow it to help you get a full night's sleep!

SLEEPING PILLS:
OTHER TIMING CONSIDERATIONS

1. If this is your first experience with a particular medication, you may wish to start on a weekend night so that you are not assessing its daytime side effects while on the job.
2. Make sure you have the potential for a reasonable night of sleep. For safety reasons you must allow time for most of the drug you are using

to clear before rising. The half-life of Ambien is relatively short, about two-and-a-half hours. Even so, after taking this medication a full night in bed, spanning at least seven hours, is recommended. The half-life of Lunesta by contrast is about six hours, so by definition half of it is still active after that same span of time. A full eight hours in bed is required for those taking Lunesta, with a reduction in dosage or switch of medication recommended if hangover effects are perceived.

3. On the other hand, don't be overly optimistic about how much more sleep pills can provide. If you typically experience less than six hours of broken sleep across nine hours in bed, and then find that with Ambien you can accumulate up to an additional hour, you should not persist in setting aside nine hours for time in bed. In fact, seven to seven-and-a-half hours may be plenty, to be extended if you start filling nearly all the allotted time with sleep, or are feeling a bit hungover when you rise.

4. Don't ask your sleeping pill to help you sleep at a vastly different time right away. If you typically get your best sleep, such as it is, from 2 A.M. into the morning, it makes more sense to take your medicine at, say, 1 A.M. and sleep better on a late schedule for a while, gradually moving sleep earlier, rather than taking it at 10:30 P.M. and experiencing broken sleep due to underlying circadian factors. Chapter 6 will

give you more effective strategies for advancing your sleep phase.

5. Unless your provider has given you other instructions, take your medicine no earlier than thirty minutes before you turn out the light. Some of you may find that it works best to just take the pill and turn in, that you are sufficiently relaxed at that point to fall asleep quickly. Others may wish to read a bit in bed, while your medicine takes effect, to continue the wind-down period that started outside the bedroom. We feel this is a reasonable departure from strict sleep hygiene rules, so long as you are looking at a printed page with a small reading lamp rather than following links on a brightly lit screen. We do not recommend remaining in your reading chair for more than thirty minutes after taking a sleeping pill. For then you will have to negotiate the transfer to bed (and perhaps a flight of stairs) while already under the drug's sway.

HOW DO **YOU** USE SLEEPING PILLS?

Even though millions of poor sleepers rely to some extent on sleeping pills, there are really only four ways they do it. The first hardly counts as usage: You may keep a bottle of pills in your medicine cabinet but rarely feel the need to take them. You might consider them an "insurance policy." Indeed, a small stash of sleep aids can provide a sense of security and confidence around the clock. Stowed safely, they work as if by magic—without the need for ingestion, and therefore without the side effects of a completed pharmacological transaction. If your day brings unexpected turmoil, if the night turns out to be truly horrendous, your pills are there for the taking. What usually happens, fortunately, is that things don't turn out so badly, and sleep arrives unaided.

The second way you might use sleeping pills is as needed. Medicine has long recognized a role for "prn" drug administration, sometimes in conjunction with other preventative medications taken daily. Usually, the decision to prescribe a particular drug on an as-needed basis is fairly straightforward, reflecting the sporadic nature of the condition being treated. For example, when an itchy rash develops, a soothing ointment is applied. When a migraine headache or an asthma attack appears despite having taken preventative measures, a "rescue medicine" may be self-administered. This puts decision making in the hands of the patient. You decide when symptoms reach the threshold for intervention.

Those of you who intermittently resort to sleep aids often base your decision on temporal factors, whether pertaining to the past, present, or future. For example, after ruefully recalling several nights of disrupted sleep, you may conclude that enough is enough; tonight you are allowing yourself some help. Or you may take stock of your present mental state and determine yourself to be way too anxious or wired to fall asleep unaided. Finally, you may be anticipating tomorrow's big presentation, or the long drive to the in-laws, and decide to take a pill rather than take chances with sleep. Whatever your choice on a given night, you trust you can get by either way. True, you probably assume you'll enjoy better sleep with a pill. However, you know you can muddle through the coming night, as well as the next day, without one.

Those of you in the third group are not so sanguine about your ability to cope without sleeping pills. You obtain a monthly supply from your provider, and then take your medication as directed, every night. As discussed at the outset of this chapter, you may or may not be satisfied with the sleep you obtain—because continuous long-term administration may well have reduced your drug's effectiveness—but at this point you are quite certain that things would go a whole lot worse at night without it.

Finally there is the fourth group, those of you in the most dire straits. Taking your pills as recommended no longer yields a tolerable amount of sleep. You find yourself doubling and even tripling the dosage in your quest for relief, with the result that you usually run out of your monthly prescription in just a couple of weeks. You spend a lot of time worrying about how you can fill the gap, and may have lined up other providers to write prescriptions either for the same or alternative sleep aids. Out of desperation, you may have felt compelled to secure a supply of pills on the street or via the internet.

If you recognize yourself in this last description, you are exhibiting classic signs of drug abuse, and should speak to your provider right away. While you have built up a tolerance for sleep aids that may mitigate their side effects even at high doses, abrupt withdrawal will likely result in severe rebound insomnia, and may be dangerous depending upon the medications you are using and their dosages. While all drug tapers should be medically supervised, it is imperative that your provider is apprised of this situation. You can eventually learn cognitive behavioral skills that, perhaps in conjunction with an alternative, monitored drug regimen, will impart adequate sleep with a lot less worry and risk.

TWO NEW WAYS TO GET OFF SLEEPING PILLS

If your use of sleeping pills falls into either of the first two groups outlined above, you and your doctor may decide that the medication is working for you as intended, and that no change of course is required. Those of you who wished to cease even sporadic usage could probably just "raise the bar" for administration to the point that you in essence joined the first group, who take comfort from their pills rather than actually taking them.

Those of you in the third and fourth groups have probably tried to get off sleeping pills many times in the past, clearly without success. As we have stressed, there are both pharmacological and psychological reasons behind your failure. The pharmacological factors are more straightforward, and may generally be addressed through a gradual taper. On the other hand, your brain's ability to trigger a relentless night of insomnia solely through anticipatory anxiety whenever you try to make do with even a reduced dosage (let alone no drug at all) calls for some wily maneuvering. Long years of experience have convinced us that trying to outsmart your own brain into sleeping is a fool's errand. It's better to try either ignorance or absurdity.

Before we get into specifics, it's important to emphasize that these strategies require you to first prepare the way, by addressing as best you can all the factors contributing to your insomnia highlighted in the other chapters. In our clinical practice, we typically introduce CBT-I interventions to regulate and consolidate sleep *prior* to collaborating with medical providers on a drug taper.

We have successfully used a method that keeps insomnia patients in the dark with regard to exactly how much medication they are using on a given night. It allows you to gradually reduce your reliance on medication while at the same time reducing the anticipatory anxiety that can so easily sabotage sleep on nights when a smaller dosage is taken. Your physician, if agreeable, would provide both a prescription of your sleep aid in a form that can be easily divided (no controlled release formulations, which do not act properly if the outer shell is breached, and no capsules full of gel or tiny particles) along with some empty capsules, of the type used in a compounding pharmacy. The other ingredient required is typically about a quarter teaspoon of sugar per capsule. Other fillers that can be used if even a small amount of regular sugar is contraindicated include the sugar alcohol mannitol, as well as milk or rice powders.

The next step is to make up a ten-night supply of medication composed of, say, eight pills at full strength embedded in the sugar-filled capsules, and two pills at half strength. You would assemble these capsules yourself to verify that the ratio is indeed as planned, but then shake all the pills in the bottle so that the dosage you take on a particular night is unknown. When this supply is depleted, a new course of medication is concocted, this time containing six full-strength pills and four pills at half strength. You would continue to substitute two more half-strength pills in subsequent batches such that in just under six weeks, your entire ten-night supply would consist of pills that are only half strength. You would then repeat the entire process, now substituting pure sugar pills (or, for an even more gradual taper, quarter-strength pills) for the half-strength pills, at the same rate of two more in each subsequent batch.

We have also found that sleeping pills can be successfully tapered with full disclosure of a given night's dosage, so long as the brain's tendency to habituate and the mind's appreciation of silliness are recruited to the effort. Under this plan, your provider again supplies sleep medication at your habitual dosage, in a divisible formulation. When ready to begin, you use a pill cutter to separate off a small portion of the pill to save for later in the taper. (Ideally you should try to remove a quarter or a third, although some pills, it is true, are hard enough to split in half without creating a powdery mess.) Under this plan it is also important to keep sleep logs throughout.

Let's say you have a round 10 mg zolpidem (Ambien) pill that you are able to split into halves and quarters. You would start the taper by alternating your regular 10 mg dose on night 1 with a 7.5 mg dose on night 2, then back to 10 mg on night 3, then 7.5 mg on night 4, and so on. The key to this plan is that *there is no adjusting of dosages allowed*. If you took 10 mg on Tuesday night, you must take 7.5 mg on Wednesday night, even if you just discovered it's going to be a big day tomorrow at work. You'll take your regular 10 mg dose again on Thursday.

During the first week or two of this alternation, you may indeed feel that you get better sleep with the slightly higher dose. While it is possible that you are sensitive to the slight pharmacological difference, it is much more likely that expectancy effects are at work. In any case, the cognitive behavioral interventions you have put into place will eventually overshadow the effects of a quarter dose of medication. At some point you will look over your recent sleep logs and realize that there is no consistent variation in sleep that can be attributed to the slightly differing dosages. *It doesn't matter which dose you take.* At that point you are ready to use 7.5 mg as your new nightly dose, which you should do for the next week or two.

Then you'll be ready to alternate 7.5 mg with 5 mg just as described above. You can see where we're going with this. One night you will be reaching for those 2.5 mg pieces you cut away earlier, and by the time you are alternating these slivers with no pill at all, the absurdity of crediting a tiny amount of medication for your better nights of sleep should be clear.

Congratulations! Whichever method you employed, you are no longer reliant on sleeping pills. You have convinced yourself you can get sleepy without them, have stopped chasing zzz's, and are gaining confidence, night by night, that sleep will find you instead.

CHAPTER SUMMARY

- Reliance on sleeping pills gives rise to diverse concerns. Some people are anxious primarily about securing their supply; they see the drugs as working just fine. Others sleep well on drugs, but are wary of their side effects and risks. Finally, some feel trapped: their sleep is not great with sleeping pills, but awful when they try to do without them.

- Regular users of sleeping pills tend to attribute any sleep they do get to the drug, rather than taking partial credit. They have what psychologists call an "external locus of control." Good sleepers, by contrast, assume an internal locus. They feel their sleep to emanate from within.

- The benefits of taking sleeping pills stem from a mix of pharmacology and psychology. They are indeed active substances, shown to produce modest increases in sleep in rigorously controlled studies. In addition, they facilitate a "handoff" in responsibility for sleep. After ingestion, users finally relax and stop trying so hard to fall off, which itself induces sleep.

- When sleeping pills lose effectiveness, neurophysiological and behavioral changes are usually to blame. The brain is very adept at habituation; most psychoactive substances produce their most dramatic effects when first introduced, and gradually lose potency. Meanwhile, poor sleep hygiene practices go uncorrected, and eventually counter the pill's diminished benefits.

- Many kinds of medication are employed as sleep aids.

Whether one would benefit you should be discussed with your healthcare provider. We see hypnotics as useful when daytime stresses are extraordinary and time-limited. Anxiolytics taken midevening set the stage for sleep while avoiding pairing a pill directly with bed. Low-dose sedating antidepressants are often used as sleep aids over longer time frames. While over-the-counter sleep aids are popular, they are not without risks, including morning hangover effects and memory problems.

- With sleep aids, timing is critical. If you typically wait until you are unable to sleep before resorting to them, you are essentially training yourself to stay awake, and increasing the risk of morning hangover. Taking a pill several hours before bed, in the hope of giving it "time to work," instead wastes its peak effectiveness, and increases the risk of falls before you turn in.

- Patients using sleep aids may be divided into four groups. The first stores pills in the medicine cabinet for "insurance." The second uses them intermittently, when waking life is particularly stressful. The third takes a pill every night, strongly believing that sleep will not appear otherwise. The fourth has grown so dependent on drugs that prescribed dosages no longer provide relief, and are often doubled up out of desperation. For those of you in the latter two groups, we offer two novel means of tapering sleep aids you might discuss with your provider.

Afterword

As we complete our work together, you hopefully now have a clear understanding why sleepiness, not sleep, is what you should really be striving for at bedtime. When you are snug in bed for the night, sleepiness is magically transformed— no longer a blight on wakefulness, it becomes the blissful portal into sleep. And unlike sleep, sleepiness is a state you can actually attain with effort—in this case the effort to change all the maladaptive thoughts, attitudes, and behaviors that have become entrenched in response to years of sleep disturbance.

Changing old ways that seem to be making the best of a bad situation is not easy. After all, your mistrust of sleep was acquired through hard experience. At this point you may feel that your sleep is beyond repair. Aggravation, anxiety, and hopelessness are understandable reactions, when you are forsaken by such a basic life function. Who could fault you for taking whatever steps you deem necessary to compensate for the loss, whether pills, naps, double espressos, oversleeping, binge-viewing, excessive bedrest, droning podcasts, or other measures? Nothing else seems to have much helped.

A key takeaway of this book is that your sleep may be temperamental, but it is not broken. Like a quirky car engine, it can still run okay if you are knowledgeable about its particular ways, and apply a little finesse. This is why we have gone into such detail when discussing what made you prone to poor sleep. This is why we have disclosed the complexities of what you are up against now, rather than promising a simple overnight fix. This is why we have laid out a number of paths to follow going forward, each leading in its own way to the threshold of sleep.

One of these paths makes sense for you. It circumvents the sleep-disruptive traits you were born with, the challenging conditions you didn't ask for. While your personal path to sleepiness may not be straightforward, or so easy to traverse, it will be well marked. We've taken pains to show you where you are heading, and what you can expect along the way.

It may take you weeks to reach your goal, maybe even months. You can do a lot of things right for a while and still not see much progress. On the other hand, you can make some mistakes along the way and still do well. Perfect adherence to all our many recommendations is not required. Just heed enough of them to start feeling sleepy at bedtime.

Finally, we are not trying to fool anyone here—we all know that being sleepy is not the same as being asleep. Sleepiness and sleep, though neighboring states, are still separated by a mysterious barrier. One last change must take place before you can drift across that moat: as you lie in bed each night, sleepy if not yet asleep, you must learn to accept that the sleepiness washing over your eyelids and your limbs, the sleepiness quieting your internal organs, the sleepiness weighing on your thoughts, is clear evidence that *you have sleep in you.*

As this core conviction grows, it will give you the confidence to stop seeking sleep elsewhere. You will cease worrying about sleep's nightly arrivals and departures; you will stop fretting over how you will ever get by tomorrow. More and more often, you'll be pleasantly surprised in the morning. Eventually, you'll come to think of yourself as an adequate sleeper, even if not the world's best. That single change of mind, together with all that you've learned in these pages, will suffice; sleep will do the rest.

Acknowledgments

Writing a book in one's free time presents quite a challenge. This volume would likely have remained just an idea if not for the encouragement of my wife, Maureen McNeil. Her ability to bring work to fruition amid the rush of daily life has long been an inspiration. I am also grateful to Jim Levine and Kerry Sparks, at Levine Greenberg Rostan Literary Agency, for their sustained support. I wish to acknowledge both my editors at Diversion Books: Randall Klein, for the deft touch and enthusiasm he brought to the project, and Lia Ottaviano, for shepherding it through to completion. I appreciate, as well, the fine production and art work done by Sarah Masterson Hally and her team. Allison Siebern, PhD; Lauren Broch, PhD; Garrick Applebee, MD; and Howard Weiss, MD generously gave of their expertise and judgment as manuscript reviewers. Will Glovinsky and Liz Bowen offered excellent advice, as fellow writers, on guiding readers through its pages. Finally, I wish to thank my patients. They have taught me much through their honesty and courage.

• • •

I called Art from the island of Samos in Greece, where I was supposed to be vacationing in August 2014, and told him we were starting on our second book. Art had received some very difficult diagnoses only five months earlier. True to form, he didn't miss a beat as he grasped the essence of the project and enthusiastically reeled off a list of issues to develop. So began the first of our many work sessions, scheduled between rounds of chemotherapy. Art relished each opportunity to talk sleep instead of illness, and, while his stamina held, he applied his prodigious conceptual ability and clinical acumen to the work.

We got about two-thirds through the first draft together. Carrying on alone stymied me for a while—after all, our partnership had spanned more than thirty years. Then Art's exhortations started to break through my loss, like a radio signal picked up from afar. What was I waiting for? Our spirited debates resumed on this mysterious channel, and I got back on task. I hope I have done Art justice, and find solace in knowing that, together once more, we may bring a measure of relief to those who are bereft of sleep.

Paul Glovinsky, PhD
New York, October 2016

Additional Resources

These books offer cognitive behavioral treatments for insomnia from the perspectives of a number of experienced practitioners:

Carney, Colleen, and Rachel Manber. 2013. *Goodnight Mind: Turn off Your Noisy Thoughts and Get a Good Night's Sleep*. Oakland, CA: New Harbinger Publications.

Edinger, Jack, and Colleen Carney. 2014. *Overcoming Insomnia: A Cognitive-Behavioral Therapy Approach: Workbook*. 2nd ed. New York: Oxford University Press.

Glovinsky, Paul, and Arthur Spielman. 2006. *The Insomnia Answer: A Personalized Program for Identifying and Overcoming the Three Types of Insomnia*. New York: Perigee.

Hauri, Peter, and Shirley Motter Linde. 1996. *No More Sleepless Nights*. Rev. ed. New York: John Wiley & Sons.

Jacobs, Gregg D. 2009. *Say Goodnight to Insomnia: The Six-*

Week, Drug-Free Program Developed at Harvard Medical School. Updated ed. New York: Holt Paperbacks.

Silberman, Stephanie A. 2009. *The Insomnia Workbook: A Comprehensive Guide to Getting the Sleep You Need.* Oakland, CA: New Harbinger Publications.

Terman, Michael, and Ian McMahon. 2012. *Chronotherapy: Resetting Your Inner Clock to Boost Mood, Alertness and Quality Sleep.* New York: Avery Books.

Two popular books covering cognitive restructuring and other aspects of cognitive behavioral therapy for depression:

Burns, David D. 2008. *Feeling Good: The New Mood Therapy.* New York: Avon Books.

Greenberger, Dennis, and Christine A. Padesky, 2016. *Mind Over Mood: Change how you feel by changing the way you think.* 2nd ed. New York: The Guilford Press.

Web-based resources for insomnia treatment:

Website of the Society of Behavioral Sleep Medicine, which maintains a roster of certified behavioral sleep medicine practitioners: www.behavioralsleep.org.

Website of the American Academy of Sleep Medicine, which includes a listing of accredited sleep disorders centers: www.aasmnet.org.

Website of the Center for Environmental Therapeutics, which provides detailed information on the use of light therapy based on the work of Michael Terman and colleagues, as well as offering light boxes and other devices for purchase: www.cet.org.

Sleepio, a web-based treatment program for insomnia developed by Colin Espie, a prominent practitioner and theorist in the field, now working with colleagues at the University of Oxford: www.sleepio.com.

The program f.lux, which removes blue light from your electronic devices in the evening, when it inhibits secretion of endogenous melatonin, can be downloaded at: www.justgetflux.com.